ONE

by

ONE

by

ONE

ONE
by
ONE
by
ONE

Making a Small Difference
Amid a Billion Problems

AARON BERKOWITZ

HarperOne
An Imprint of HarperCollinsPublishers

HarperOne

FIRST EDITION

Designed by SBI Book Arts

Library of Congress Cataloging-in-Publication Data

Names: Berkowitz, Aaron, 1978– author.
Title: One by one by one : making a small difference amid a billion
    problems / Aaron Berkowitz.
Description: New York, NY : HarperOne, 2020 | Includes bibliographical
    references.
Identifiers: LCCN 2019032512 (print) | LCCN 2019032513 (ebook) | ISBN
    9780062964212 (hardcover) | ISBN 9780062966520 | ISBN 9780062980618 |
    ISBN 9780062964250 (ebook)
Subjects: LCSH: Berkowitz, Aaron, 1978– | Partners in Health (Organization)
    | Neurologists—United States—Biography. |
    Brain—Tumors—Patients—Haiti. | Poor—Medical care—Haiti. | Medical
    care, Cost of—Haiti.
Classification: LCC RD592.9.B47 A3 2020 (print) | LCC RD592.9.B47 (ebook)
    | DDC 617.4/8092 [B]—dc23
LC record available at https://lccn.loc.gov/2019032512
LC ebook record available at https://lccn.loc.gov/2019032513

20 21 22 23 24 LSC 10 9 8 7 6 5 4 3 2 1

In memory of my father,

who taught me to be good and do good

To Michelle, Anne, Martineau, Ian,

Hermide, Kerling, Père Eddy, and François,

my partners in health

To Nina,

my partner in life

Hallie had been working to save lives. Not everything all at once, as Amy and so many others believed, but one by one by one . . . No impulse to reinvent the world from the bottom up, no acts of revolutionary defiance, but a commitment to doing good in the broken world she belonged to, a plan to spend her life helping others, which was not a political act so much as a religious act, a religion without religion or dogma, a faith in the value of the one and the one and the one . . . and while Amy and a host of others would have argued that people were sick because society was sick and helping them adjust to a sick society would only make them worse, Hallie would have answered, Please, go ahead and improve society if you can, but meanwhile people are suffering, and I have a job to do.

—*Paul Auster, 4321*

Our mission is to provide a preferential option for the poor in health care. By establishing long-term relationships with sister organizations based in settings of poverty, Partners In Health strives to achieve two overarching goals: to bring the benefits of modern medical science to those most in need of them and to serve as an antidote to despair.

We draw on the resources of the world's leading medical and academic institutions and on the lived experience of the world's poorest and sickest communities. At its root, our mission is both medical and moral. It is based on solidarity, rather than charity alone.

When our patients are ill and have no access to care, our team of health professionals, scholars, and activists will do whatever it takes to make them well—just as we would do if a member of our own families or we ourselves were ill.

—*Partners In Health, mission statement*

ONE
by
ONE
by
ONE

1

I present to you patient Janel, a 23-year-old male student with no prior medical history, born and currently living in Savanette, presenting for evaluation of headaches evolving over several months, a sense of vertigo when he stands, and difficulty walking.

So began an email that would intertwine the lives of Dr. Martineau Louine, the patient he described, and me. Most patients in need of neurologic care in Haiti go to primary care doctors like Martineau. Primary care doctors in Haiti can't simply refer patients to a neurologist the way they would in the US or other wealthy countries, since the only neurologist in Haiti—one for a country of more than ten million citizens—practices in the capital city of Port-au-Prince.

Port-au-Prince is only about ninety miles from Savanette, but the trip takes close to four hours. Much of the journey is on dirt roads that become impassable mud in the rainy season. The rest of the way is on paved but treacherous winding mountain roads, all the more treacherous when riding packed into the back of a pickup-truck taxi called a *taptap*, or balanced in groups of two or three on the back of a motorcycle behind the driver. The cost of transportation to make this trip—let alone the cost of an appointment with a specialist—is beyond the means of most people in Haiti. More than half the population lives on less than two dollars a day, and about a quarter on less than one dollar a day. So patients go to the closest doctor they can find. In poor, remote rural communities like Savanette, that may be a young doctor who has just finished medical school, practicing alone and without supervision—a doctor who has gone to medical school in a country with no neurologists to teach them about the diagnosis and treatment of neurologic conditions like stroke, seizure, or Parkinson's disease, let alone how to approach a more complex patient like Janel.

When I received Martineau's email about Janel in September 2014, I was just a few months out of my neurology residency training and had recently begun my first job as a neurologist at Brigham and Women's Hospital—Brigham for short—in Boston. At Brigham, I'm one of more than 100 neurologists on staff, and Brigham is one of several hospitals with large neurology departments in Boston, a city with a population of less than 700,000. One of my Brigham colleagues who worked in Haiti had asked me if I could help provide neurology training for Haitian doctors through the Boston-based non-governmental organization Partners In Health (known in the field as PIH). Founded by global health luminaries Paul Farmer, Ophelia Dahl, and Jim Yong Kim, PIH had begun its pioneering work providing healthcare to the world's poorest patients in Haiti, later expanding to work in Peru, Rwanda, Malawi, Mexico, Lesotho, Russia, Navajo Nation, Liberia, and Sierra Leone.

So I started going to Haiti to teach neurology for two weeks at a time, first yearly, then a few times each year. Martineau had identified himself as an eager and skilled collaborator. He began asking that all patients with neurologic conditions who came to PIH's recently opened Hôpital Universitaire de Mirebalais—the largest hospital in central Haiti—be referred to him. When I was in Haiti working with PIH, Martineau and I saw patients together. In between visits, he emailed me about patients he found challenging to diagnose or treat, like Janel.

Martineau's email continued:

> On physical examination, the patient had increased
> reflexes most notable in the lower extremities. There were
> trembling movements of his right arm and right leg that
> affected his walking. The tremor in his right hand affected
> his coordination when he moved his finger from his nose to
> my hand.

Martineau had attached a shaky one-and-a-half-minute cell phone video to his email. In the video, Janel is sitting on an examination table, his hands resting on his lap. Only his torso and legs are visible. He's dressed in a white button-down shirt with thin vertical purple stripes, dark blue pants, and shiny black dress shoes that dangle motionless over a white tile floor. An electronic monitor beeps continuously in the background from another clinic room. Martineau's slender arms enter the frame in a starched white dress shirt, holding his reflex hammer. His stethoscope dangles from around his neck, swinging back and forth between his arms like a pendulum as he tests Janel's reflexes. *"Lage men an, lage men an,"* Martineau says ("Relax your hands, relax your hands") as he hits each elbow crease in turn with his reflex hammer, sending Janel's hands leaping off his lap. Then Martineau hits just below Janel's kneecaps, causing his legs to kick out briskly. In the last moments of the video, Martineau asks Janel to reach his hands forward. A subtle, rapid tremor emerges in Janel's right hand, making it quiver briefly like a hummingbird's wing. Then it stops. "Okay," Martineau says, and the video ends.

For neurologists, the physical examination holds important clues to the cause of a patient's symptoms. While the stethoscope allows doctors to listen to the activities of the heart and lungs, it's the patterns of weakness, abnormal movements, reflexes, and other elements of the physical examination that neurologists observe to determine the precise site of disease within the nervous system: is the problem in the brain, the spinal cord, the nerves, the muscles? The jumpy reflexes Martineau demonstrated in the video were a clue that his patient's problem was in the central nervous system—the brain or spinal cord. The tremor that appeared with movement and disappeared with rest suggested dysfunction of the back of the brain in a part called the cerebellum.

During my first visits to Haiti, the bedside examination was all we had in neurology. Lab testing was limited, and the single CT scanner in the capital city was too expensive and too far away for most patients to access. My colleagues and I struggled to try to help many patients for whom we felt that if only we had a CT scan or an MRI, we might be able to figure out what was wrong and how to treat them. Examining a patient might lead us to conclude that there was a problem in the brain, but what was it? A stroke? An infection? A tumor? Without a scan, it was often impossible to determine.

This is the reality for many doctors and their patients in low-income countries, where there are an average of 32 CT scanners per 100 million population, more than 100 times fewer than in high-income countries. Many of these CT scanners are broken. And even where there are CT scanners that work, they are often inaccessible to most patients due to the cost or distance necessary to travel to them.

Haiti's 2010 earthquake led, albeit indirectly, to the country's first publicly available CT scanner in 2013. The earthquake devastated Haiti's overpopulated capital of Port-au-Prince, killing hundreds of thousands of people under the rubble of poorly constructed buildings and displacing more than a million people who lost their homes. Haiti's largest public hospital and nursing school were among the estimated 25,000 non-residential buildings that were damaged or destroyed. The nursing school was in session when it collapsed, ending the lives of a generation of future nurses and the teachers training them. As part of a "building back better" campaign drawing on the extraordinary outpouring of generosity toward Haiti after the earthquake—over half of US families donated—PIH built Hôpital Universitaire de Mirebalais.

Called HUM for short, it's a three-hundred-bed, solar-powered public hospital with modern operating rooms, an intensive care unit, and, most important to a neurologist, a CT scanner.

The arrival of the CT scanner in Haiti allowed me to imagine what it must have been like when this technology first became widely available in the 1970s. Before CT scans, learning to perform brain autopsies was an essential component of a neurologist's training—aspiring neurologists learned by diagnosing patients after death whom they couldn't diagnose in life. How exciting it must have felt the first time neurologists used CT scans to peer behind the curtain at the brain itself while the patient was still alive. This is something we now take for granted in most of the world. Not in Haiti. With so many patients whose neurologic illnesses previously remained undiagnosed medical mysteries, the CT scanner at HUM was similarly revolutionary for us. It was a great leap forward in our ability to provide neurologic care in Haiti, despite still being many decades behind most other countries.

Martineau had gotten a CT scan of Janel's brain and sent the file to me. I tapped the arrows on my computer keyboard to scroll through the gray images of the brain set against a black background. I'd looked at thousands of CT scans during the eighty-hour weeks of my recently completed residency. But this CT scan was unlike anything I'd ever seen. The ventricles—hollow cavities deep within the brain—were filled with a mass of abnormal tissue. It was enormous, about the size of a tennis ball. It was complex, its contour bulging out wildly in all directions, compressing and distorting the surrounding brain structures. It was described in the radiologist's report as "lobulated," "exophytic," and "cystic": multilobed, outwardly growing, and containing a fluid-filled component.

It was the largest brain tumor I'd ever seen.

I read Martineau's email again. It said Janel was a student, age twenty-three. I presumed that meant he was in college, so his cognition must not have been affected yet by the tumor. I watched the video again. Janel was sitting on the examination table, which he would have presumably had to climb onto, suggesting he had good strength and coordination. How could he have been so mildly affected with just a tremor, a little trouble walking, and brisk reflexes? I went back to the CT scan, amazed at the size and extent of the mass. If he had only minimal symptoms, maybe it was a very slow-growing tumor and his brain had somehow compensated for its intrusive but initially indolent presence. Since he was only twenty-three years old, maybe it had been there since childhood, but without a CT scanner available until recently, it had been impossible to figure out why he developed progressive neurologic symptoms.

Martineau's email concluded:

What can we do for this patient?

I wasn't sure how to respond to him. Without surgery to remove the tumor, his patient would become progressively disabled and die. But there are no neurosurgeons in Haiti trained to perform complex brain tumor surgery. Even if there were, not even the brand-new modern operating rooms at HUM have the necessary high-tech equipment to safely perform such a surgery. And no place in Haiti has the resources necessary to provide specialized postoperative care for a patient after the deepest recesses of the brain are manipulated.

Had Janel been born just a two-hour plane ride away in the US—still far shorter than the drive from his home to Port-au-Prince—he would have never ended up with a tumor so advanced as to require such a complex intervention. He would have had a scan, a diagnosis, and surgery years ago when he first developed symptoms and the tumor was much smaller and could have been more easily treated.

Working in Haiti for two years, I had seen awful things. Patients with untreated epilepsy who were covered in bruises and burns from seizures that shook them to the ground or into a cooking fire. Patients with severe meningitis (an infection of the brain's linings) who arrived too late for treatment and died of a disease easily treated in most other countries—and in many cases preventable by vaccine.

For patients with epilepsy, we could get their seizures under control with medications available in Haiti. Though the delays before appropriate treatment were often beyond anything I'd seen in the US, we could help many epileptic patients return to normal lives. For patients presenting late in the course of an illness like meningitis, there wasn't much we could do: the setting and its limited access to healthcare left us powerless to effectively intervene by the time the patients made it to us.

My colleagues in other medical specialties talked about patients they saw in Haiti with conditions that could have been instantly and easily treated by surgery in the US but proved devastatingly disabling or even fatal without adequate resources in Haiti. Yet as a neurologist in Haiti, I didn't think I had ever found myself in a situation in which I said, "If only I could get this patient to the US right now, I could make a big save."

Sadly, even in my practice in the US, big saves in neurology are generally few and far between. We can treat the pain of migraines, the seizures of epilepsy, the shaking and stiffness of Parkinson's. We can reduce the debilitating flares of multiple sclerosis and rehabilitate a patient after a stroke or head trauma. We can improve our patients' quality of life, but rarely do we cure them of their underlying disease. Even when we make an impact, it's usually not by means of high-adrenaline big saves like the ones made by our colleagues in trauma surgery or heart transplant surgery or emergency medicine. Sometimes, with diseases like ALS or Alzheimer's, we're powerless to do more than try to ease the suffering of our patients and their families as they face the disease's inevitable, tragic progression. When I was a medical student and told one of my surgery professors that I was interested in neurology, he scoffed, "Diagnose and adios—that's no fun." It's an exaggeration, of course, but diagnostics in neurology have always run ahead of treatments.

Looking back and forth between Martineau's email, Janel's CT scan, and the video of this otherwise healthy young patient, I saw the potential for a big save for the first time, not just in my work in Haiti but in the early days of my career as a doctor. Without treatment, progressive disability, suffering, and untimely death awaited this young man. But if I could somehow get him to the US for surgery to have the tumor removed, maybe he could be spared the loss of his walking, his thinking, and ultimately himself.

If anyone could help find a solution, it was my colleague and friend Dr. Michelle Morse. A brilliant young internal medicine doctor at Brigham with a tireless commitment to global health equity, Michelle cofounded a nonprofit organization called EqualHealth before she had even finished her residency. She rapidly rose through the ranks of PIH to become the deputy chief medical officer for their twelve-hospital network in Haiti and was part of the team that got HUM up and running. When I had reached out early in my residency to everyone I had met who was involved in global health to ask how a neurologist might help, Michelle was the first to reply, insisting that Haiti needed me most. Within a month, she had set me up on my first trip. When I saw her in Haiti I actually thought she was Haitian—she spoke Haitian Creole fluently, right down to slang expressions, proverbs, and even the facial expressions that accompanied them.

Michelle somehow manages to balance a radical critique of the inequities in healthcare with optimism that change is possible. Rather than try to change people's minds through argument, she leads by example. When a colleague in Boston asked her to speak to a group of doctors and trainees on bias and diversity, she lamented to me, "Of course ask one of the only African American doctors on the faculty to talk about diversity!" But to her colleague, she said, "Sure, but it won't be a PowerPoint, and it won't be just one session." Instead of giving a lecture, she brought patients to tell their own stories of discrimination they faced in the healthcare system in an eye-opening, purposefully uncomfortable, but ultimately redemptive session.

I called Michelle and was surprised when she picked up the phone. She was always coming and going between the PIH sites—Haiti, Liberia, Rwanda, Malawi. I was used to getting her voicemail, which simply said, "If you have received this message, I am probably out of the country, but you can reach me by email." I told her I had heard from Martineau about an otherwise healthy young man in Haiti with an operable brain tumor causing relatively minimal deficits. Did she think we could get this patient to the US for care? If so, how?

"You're thinking about this the right way," she began. "These are the horrific inequities we see in places like Haiti. But in cases like this, we can go beyond them. What's his name?"

"Janel," I said.

"We need to get Janel to the US," she said firmly.

We plotted the course. With its modern operating rooms, HUM had become a focal point for volunteer surgeons offering to serve in Haiti, including several groups of neurosurgeons. Michelle and I agreed that Janel's surgery would be too complex and risky to perform in Haiti, but she suggested we reach out to these neurosurgeons about his case. She hoped they might respond by proposing to bring the patient to one of their hospitals.

I sent an email and the scans to the neurosurgeons Michelle had mentioned. They agreed that the case required surgical expertise and equipment not available in Haiti. Given these resource limitations, they felt that a palliative approach should be offered. They suggested treating the excess fluid buildup in the brain that the tumor was causing by implanting a VP shunt—a system of plastic and rubber tubing connecting the brain's ventricles (the V in VP) to the abdomen (specifically the peritoneum, the P in VP). Implanting a VP shunt is a relatively quick and minor procedure compared to brain tumor surgery, and one that could be performed in Haiti. But this would do nothing about the tumor.

With a palliative approach, the neurosurgeons were proposing to treat one consequence of the disease, but not the disease itself. In other words—my disappointed, angry, PIH-inspired version of their words— provide care that is better than nothing but still let Janel worsen and die just because of where he happened to be born.

Would it be possible, I inquired in a follow-up email to the neuro- surgeons, to consider bringing the patient to one of their hospitals for surgery? The neurosurgeons wrote back that they disagreed with trying to do this for several reasons. First, they felt that bringing this patient abroad for care would be unsustainable since there was no guarantee that this could be offered to the next brain tumor patient who might arrive at HUM. Second, they thought treating the patient wouldn't be cost- effective—how could we justify hundreds of thousands of dollars' worth of care for one patient when that money could be used to help so many other patients with lower-cost illnesses? Finally, they were concerned the surgery would be too high-risk, with the potential for the patient to worsen afterward, even if performed in an optimal high-resource setting. The neurosurgeons reiterated their recommendation to pursue a pallia- tive approach by implanting a VP shunt, but not touching the tumor.

Sustainability. Cost-effectiveness. These considerations may be well- intentioned on a policy level, but they break down when faced with a patient in front of you. True, we likely wouldn't be able to help every patient who needed brain surgery in Haiti. But why should that pre- vent us from trying to help Janel? True, for the potential hundreds of thousands of dollars that would go into this one patient's treatment— surgery, intensive care, and radiation and chemotherapy if the tumor turned out to be malignant—we could vaccinate an entire region of Haiti against deadly childhood infections. We could probably even build a whole new hospital in Haiti. But try explaining that trade-off to Janel. What would be the point of building more hospitals if they would never be able to help *him*? If we extend life for the world's poorest by providing vaccines and other aspects of primary healthcare, what do we tell our patients when they develop more complex conditions, like brain tumors?

Paul Farmer—one of PIH's founders and current leaders—has described the struggle to serve those right in front of you while simultaneously working to reduce the longer-term risk of others ending up in front of you as the chief tension of PIH's work.

With Janel right in front of us, it actually didn't seem like that much of a tension to me. I knew I couldn't come up with a sustainable, cost-effective solution that would solve enormous problems like global poverty and inequitable access to modern healthcare—I would have to leave that to the Paul Farmers of the world. But as a doctor, couldn't I try to help this one patient?

About 4 billion people lack access to basic healthcare, let alone the type of advanced healthcare that patients like Janel require. That's more than half the world's population. It's an astronomical number, 4,000,000,000. We count stars in billions; Earth is 4.5 billion years old. It's an overwhelming number—it would take more than 120 years to count to 4 billion at a rate of one number per second. But it's a real number. A real number of real people. Patients like Janel remind us that overwhelming global statistics are composed of individuals, each with hopes and dreams, family and friends, and a right to live a healthy life free of disease.

Every billion is made up of a billion ones.

PIH describes its work as being based on solidarity rather than charity alone. Charity is necessary, of course: those who have more should help those who have less. But charity means us giving to them, to some abstract all. Solidarity redefines this relationship. It invites all of us to share with each other, because we are each part of the same all.

The final phrase of PIH's mission statement illuminates what's at stake when adopting this solidarity-based approach to medicine:

When our patients are ill and have no access to care, our team of health professionals, scholars, and activists will do whatever it takes to make them well—just as we would do if a member of our own families or we ourselves were ill.

What would it mean for me to try to do whatever it takes to make Janel well, whatever it takes as if he were a member of my own family, whatever it takes as if he were me myself?

Aspiring to live up to this mission statement, I felt compelled to try to get Janel the care he needed, to bring the benefits of modern medicine to him, or him to the benefits of modern medicine. But the neurosurgeons we had written to clearly thought this wasn't a good idea—unsustainable, not cost-effective, too complicated. Should I throw up my hands at the inequity that's a much larger problem than Janel alone, turn a blind eye to his bad luck, and focus instead on helping patients in simpler situations with more straightforward solutions? Or should I choose solidarity over sustainability, compassion over cost-effectiveness?

I chose solidarity. I decided to try to do whatever it took to help Janel, to commit to this credo, to make this mission statement my mission. Did I make the right decision? This book explores that question, telling the story of what happened when I stepped from the realm of inspiring principles into the reality of taking action. It's a story of triumphs, tragedies, and the confusing spaces in between as I attempted to bridge the gap between the rich-world medical metropolis of Boston and one of the world's poorest regions in rural Haiti. It's about what I learned and grappled with as I strived to do what I thought was the right thing and struggled to figure out the right way to do it.

By choosing solidarity with Janel and other patients in Haiti, I witnessed their extraordinary bravery, courage, and faith as they faced debilitating neurologic disease in the midst of dire poverty. By choosing solidarity with doctors in Haiti like Martineau, I found inspiration in their humble heroism as they advocated for their patients to get the care they desperately needed, even when it didn't exist in their country. And by choosing solidarity with my colleagues in Boston to do whatever it took to help our patients in Haiti, I learned how a few individuals working together might just be able to make a small difference in those big billions, one by one by one.

2

It didn't look like we were going to be able to convince anyone in the group of neurosurgeons we had emailed to bring Janel to one of their hospitals for surgery. But Michelle didn't let them off so easily. She wrote them an email to, as she put it, "help them understand why their answer was the wrong answer."

> This is not the first nor the last time we will come across these kinds of heartbreaking patients, and continue to try to find a way where there is no way, because we know that we can help. True, this is not a "sustainable" approach, but when the patients arrive in front of us, it is hard to not do everything possible to help that one patient. Sustainable health care in Haiti will take decades . . . I understand wanting to stay in the scope, but do also know that with this work, we have to be flexible . . . I can't predict what cases are coming our way, but do appreciate our ongoing conversations about these really tough ethical challenges . . . I do also think that as we find these patients, we should do the best we can. We have been successful in getting some patients to the US for surgery, and I think it's worth a serious try for this patient.

The neurosurgeons didn't reply.

Disappointed but determined, we decided to try our own hospital, Brigham and Women's. Although I had spent the previous four years training there, I had just undergone the humbling transition from being one of the most senior trainees in neurology to being the most junior staff physician. As a new faculty member in my first months of practice, I wasn't sure what the neurosurgeons would make of an email query from me, or if they would even read it among the backup of emails they must have after spending the entire day—and sometimes the entire night—operating. To get our neurosurgeon colleagues and the hospital on board with offering free care to Janel, I needed some higher-level backing. I decided to present the case at morning report.

Morning report in the Brigham neurology department takes place at 7:30 a.m. every weekday. Neurology residents, students, and faculty cram around a big conference table in a small room to discuss patients who had been seen the night before in the emergency room or who were being cared for on the ward. At the head of the table sits Dr. Martin A. Samuels, the chair of the department for nearly thirty years. A young seventy, tall and slender, with thin-rimmed spectacles and an impressive collection of bow ties, Dr. Samuels fits the visual description of most people's stereotype of a Harvard professor. And so does his CV. He has quite literally written the book on neurology, coauthoring the encyclopedic 1,600-page textbook that is considered the go-to reference in our field. The awards and honorary degrees he has accumulated over his illustrious career fill every inch of wall space in his office and spill out into the hallways beyond it. But he is humble, humorous, unassuming, and down-to-earth. His office has a piano, a tissue dispenser that dispenses tissues out of the nostrils of a large nose, and several framed photographs of Freddy, his feisty Norfolk terrier. Not one for hierarchy, he goes by Marty. It was Marty who offered me a job at Brigham and provided me with the flexibility, freedom, mentorship, and support to work part of the year in Haiti. My hope was that if I could get him interested in Janel's case at morning report, he might help me approach the neurosurgeons and the hospital administration.

When the residents finished presenting the cases they had seen over the prior night, I asked if I could get the group's advice on a case

from Haiti. I gave the brief story and described the physical examination from Martineau's video. Then we turned out the lights to look
at the CT scan on a large monitor that hung on the wall of the conference room. As the enormous tumor came into view, faculty members, residents, and students gasped and whispered in the darkness.
Nobody had seen anything like it.

"Can anything be done for him in Haiti?" one of my faculty colleagues asked me.

"Unfortunately . . ." I began.

"You have to bring him here for neurosurgery!" Marty interrupted
enthusiastically. Others around the table nodded slowly in agreement,
their faces palely illuminated by the digital light from the projected
images of Janel's tumor.

Success! I thought excitedly. But I suppressed a smile and soberly
said, "I'm going to try."

Having Marty's support would go a long way. He is a legendary
figure at Brigham due to his long tenure as a charismatic chairman,
renowned clinician and educator, and admired colleague. I decided
to see if he could help me get a Brigham neurosurgeon interested in
Janel's case. Approaching him after morning report as he opened the
door from the conference room to his adjoining office, I asked him
which Brigham neurosurgeon he thought I should contact.

"Ian Dunn," he replied. "He's one of our top brain tumor surgeons.
He does all the most complex cases with impressive results. Good guy
too. Tell him I suggested you write to him. Keep up the great work
you're doing in Haiti." He smiled and disappeared into his office, and
I ran to my office and wrote an email to Ian Dunn about Janel with a
well-placed reference to Marty Samuels in the opening line.

It worked. Just twenty minutes after I'd sent my email, Ian replied:

> It's an impressive scan. I think it is definitely worth trying
> to get him here for a definitive MRI and likely attempt at
> resection. While large and deep, it does seem to be readily

distinguishable from the thalamus. Obviously we are happy to help in any way.

Success again! was my first thought. But my second thought was about the thalamus. Situated centrally and deep within the brain, the thalamus is a crucial structure for consciousness. All modalities of perception—visual, auditory, tactile—are processed there en route to the cortex on the outer surface of the brain, where they rise to the level of conscious awareness. Important circuits for movement and coordination make critical connections in this vital structure. Even small strokes or hemorrhages in the thalamus can leave patients comatose or severely disabled.

Suddenly it hit me. In my eagerness to go for a big save and in my knee-jerk reaction against arguments of cost-effectiveness and sustainability when a person's life was on the line, I had neglected to consider the final point of trepidation raised by the neurosurgeons Michelle and I had emailed: the high risk of surgery. I was asking a neurosurgeon to remove a tumor dangerously close to a structure essential for conscious existence. And I had never even met the patient.

I realized queasily that I was entering the type of situation that caused doctors to be accused of "playing God." I would be making decisions for Janel that could have life-or-death consequences. At first, bringing him to the US had seemed like a no-brainer: a twenty-three-year-old healthy student with a brain tumor who could be treated should be treated. But this same treatment that could prevent him from getting worse—or at best make him better if we weren't several years too late—also held the risk of severe or even fatal complications.

As a neurologist, I had never had the "playing God" feeling I imagined some doctors experience. When I was a medical student, I saw cardiac surgeons stop a patient's heart and then start it beating again. I watched neurosurgeons saw open the skull to reveal the brain, pulsating and bloody and glistening under the bright lights of the operating room. I imagined that even the most humble surgeons must find it hard not to feel as though they're playing God when they shake hands with patients before and after they cut them open, handle their internal organs, and sew them back together with those same hands. Thinking through Janel's case, I began to have a sense of what a weighty feeling that must be.

I discussed the situation over breakfast in the hospital cafeteria with a colleague who was also involved in global health work.

"Every time . . ." He trailed off wistfully, slowly shaking his head as he looked beyond me at the flurry of hospital staff caffeinating at the coffee machines.

"Every time we tried to buck the system to make something miraculous happen abroad that we couldn't accomplish in the field . . ." He trailed off again.

"Every time . . . Every time, something terrible happened," he finally said.

My colleague told me about a young girl who developed failure of one of her heart valves. He and his colleagues knew she would die without a valve replacement surgery, but the surgery couldn't be done in the country where they worked. Seeing the potential for a big save and trying to avoid a senseless death from a treatable disease, they found a cardiac surgeon abroad willing to do the surgery. But the mechanical valve the surgeon needed to implant required that the young girl be on a blood thinner medication for the rest of her life, which required frequent blood tests to monitor its effects. Somehow my colleague and his group not only got the young girl abroad for surgery but also figured out how to provide the medication and monitoring over the long term. The patient had successful heart surgery and was celebrated as a huge triumph.

Then she died suddenly. The cause was a fatal brain hemorrhage, a complication of the blood thinning medication my colleague had worked so hard to obtain.

"We felt terrible." He looked down at his steaming coffee. Then he looked up at me. "It was the 'right thing to do,' you know?" he said, making quotes in the air with his hands. "And we thought we had crossed every *t* and dotted every *i*, and then . . ." He looked down again and swallowed hard. "Somehow it feels like when you try to intervene against the natural course of things . . . well . . . maybe you can't. We stopped trying to do this sort of thing to maintain our focus on building local capacity."

Janel's surgery would carry enormous risks: worsening disability, coma, even death. As a neurologist, I regularly discussed the potential risks and benefits of surgery and other treatments with my patients. From conversations that had gone better or worse—for the patients or for me—I had developed a sort of script that seemed to work most of the time. "While some patients in your situation say they would take any risk for the chance of improvement," I would say, "other patients prefer not to be so aggressive, to accept the situation and let nature take its course." Then I would pause. If there was no response, no identification with one of these extremes, I would continue, "But most patients fall somewhere in between. Where are you in this decision process at the moment, and what questions can I answer?"

With patients in Boston, I felt we at least shared a somewhat common frame of reference. People had friends or family who'd had surgery, maybe even brain surgery. They'd heard of a coma on TV or in movies, and had perhaps even seen it in their own loved ones. They came to these discussions with some experience and background—and therefore some intuition—about how much fear and hope to have.

But how would this look to Janel, a twenty-three-year-old in rural Haiti? In the remote, destitute region where he lived, nobody would have gotten neurosurgery, nobody would have had a television to watch a show in which someone got brain surgery or lived for a prolonged period in a coma. How would he balance these abstract risks against an extraordinary faith in *doktè blan*? "White doctors" is the literal translation of *doktè blan*, though the word *blan* in Haitian Creole is used to describe all foreigners whether or not their skin is white. Many *doktè blan* come to Haiti on mission trips each year to offer surgeries not otherwise possible there—interventions that can appear miraculous to local communities. Not only would we be speaking as *doktè blan*; we would be offering surgery *lòt bò a*—on "the other side," as the US is often referred to in Creole—widely seen as a land of medical miracles.

We could ask Martineau, Janel's doctor, to explain to him that even in the best-case scenario, surgery might only prevent him from getting worse rather than make him better, and that there would be a significant risk of surgery making things worse. But would these subtleties of risk and benefit resonate, or would Janel be biased by belief in a miracle when Martineau mentioned *doktè blan* and *lòt bò a*?

To provide Martineau with the best information for his discussion with Janel, I wrote to Ian again to get his sense of the surgery's risks:

> Do you think it is reasonable to say that based on the CT scan, aside from the risks inherent in any major neurosurgical procedure, that this tumor appears potentially highly amenable to surgical therapy, although of course the prognosis beyond this will depend on what type of tumor it turns out to be? My colleagues in Haiti will have to present all of this carefully to the patient so he and his family can balance the risks and benefits of leaving his country for a major surgery.

A man of few words, Ian replied:

> I agree with your comments. MRI will be a bit more helpful in saying that more forcefully.

An MRI provides a much more detailed view of brain anatomy and pathology than a CT scan. If we could get free care for Janel in Boston, he would have an MRI after he arrived, both to give us a better understanding of what type of tumor it may be and for Ian to plan his surgical approach. But what if we brought Janel to Boston based only on the results of the CT scan and the MRI revealed that the tumor was invading the brain rather than just pushing against it, making it inoperable? This outcome not only would be deeply disappointing to Janel but also could jeopardize future attempts to bring patients from Haiti to Boston. If we went through all of the trouble to get Janel to Boston only to send him home after an MRI, it would look like we didn't really know what we were doing.

An MRI center had recently opened in Haiti, and for about seven hundred dollars we could get Janel an MRI. Although this was necessary before making any further decisions, I worried that even the MRI could provide false hope for him and his family since an expensive and high-tech test was being offered for free. For a few weeks I'd been involved in email chains with Michelle, Martineau, Ian, and others about whether getting Janel to the US was even possible, and I felt bad that we hadn't yet brought the patient and his family into the discussion. But we wanted to be able to provide as much information as possible to help them make an informed decision.

I called Martineau.

"It is a very complicated situation, isn't it?" Martineau asked, cutting right to the heart of the matter after we exchanged greetings.

We went over everything we had been discussing by email. The only treatment for this enormous tumor would be surgery, but the surgery wasn't possible in Haiti. It would have to be performed abroad, and it was a high-risk surgery. There was even a risk of his patient dying in Boston, far away from his home and family. I asked Martineau if he could make sure that Janel and his family understood these risks before we proceeded any further toward trying to get him to the US. I told Martineau about my concern that it could be hard for Janel and his family to fully grasp these risks because of any blind faith they might have in a free surgery performed in the US.

"I don't mean to imply that they wouldn't understand," I said. "I just worry that . . . Well, as you said, it's complicated."

"In general," Martineau explained to me, "people who come from

the rural areas may seem simple since they do not have access to education. But they understand. There are certain words, and once those
words resonate in their ears, they have an idea. For example, when you
say 'operation,' this word is heavy with consequence for them. It in-
vokes fear. The doctor is going to take a knife to you. So they know
there's a lot of risk. They know once there is an indication for an operation, in general, there is no going back."

In addition to being a brilliant physician and colleague, Martineau
had always helped me understand the patients we saw together in Haiti
and the context in which they lived. He offered to present everything to
Janel and let us know what he thought.

A few days later, Martineau wrote to me and Michelle.

> Unfortunately, the patient has no family to support him. He
> was abandoned by his mother some time ago and is now
> cared for in a church, where the pastor provides housing,
> food, and transportation fees to send him to the hospital. The
> congregation and patient are ready to take the risk of surgical
> intervention presuming total and unconditional financial
> support by the US hospital, because the patient has no family
> in Haiti or in the US. So now it is up to us to determine if we
> can take on all of these responsibilities.

Sadly, abandonment of sick children is not uncommon in Haiti.
Infants are sometimes left in the hospital after delivery, because the
parents either can't afford to take care of them or think better-off
hospital staff might adopt them and provide a better life for the child
than the parents could. Once, a severely disabled teenager with cere-
bral palsy was simply left on the doorstep of the HUM rehabilitation
ward, bedbound and unable to speak, only able to writhe and scream.
The rehabilitation team never figured out where he had come from. No
long-term care facility in Haiti would accept him, and so he has lived
on the rehabilitation ward ever since.

I was both saddened by the story of Janel's abandonment and impressed by the extraordinary commitment of his church to take him in and support him. But I worried that a young man with no mother or father would raise a red flag for hospital administrators in Boston. They would be concerned about whether there was a safe and sustainable plan for the patient after he returned to Haiti, especially if he suffered a complication of surgery that made him worse.

Although the news of Janel's circumstances worried me, it didn't seem to bother Michelle. Her one-line reply to Martineau was emblematic of her tireless commitment to helping the poorest patients irrespective of potential structural barriers:

> Agree, very unfortunate situation but even more reason why we should help!

Martineau organized the MRI, and Michelle and I pitched in the seven-hundred-dollar cost to make sure we wouldn't be waiting for budget approvals or other administrative delays in securing the funds.

One month after Martineau had originally contacted me about Janel, he got his MRI. It confirmed that the large tumor was arising in the ventricles and compressing the surrounding brain structures but not invading them. I sent the images to Ian. His response was what I was beginning to recognize as his usual mix of terse and definitive neurosurgical precision:

> I would definitely offer surgery here. Thanks for sending the images and involving me.

Since we now had confirmation that surgery would be offered at Brigham and that the patient was willing to accept the risks, Michelle and I began reaching out to hospital administrators to ask about the logistics. Our administrative colleagues at Brigham outlined the following steps: fill out hospital paperwork applying for free care based on the patient's financial situation, obtain a cost estimate of the operation from the neurosurgery administration, apply for outside funding to help offset the hospital's costs, and develop a clear plan for where the patient would go when he was discharged from the hospital before he returned to Haiti.

In order to provide free care, the hospital required documented proof that the patient couldn't pay, such as bank records. This step was simple: we explained to the hospital administration that Janel was so poor he didn't even have a bank account.

The cost of Janel's surgery and perioperative care was estimated at $157,000. But many types of brain tumors require treatment with radiation and chemotherapy to reduce the risk of the tumor recurring. We presented Janel's case at a Brigham brain tumor board—a conference where all practitioners involved in the care of patients with tumors assemble to discuss cases: oncologists, radiation oncologists, surgeons, pathologists, social workers, nurses, case managers. Although nobody at the meeting had ever seen a tumor of this size, its location and radiologic characteristics suggested a few possibilities as to what type of tumor it could be. The group agreed that any of the possibilities would likely require nearly two months of radiation after surgery. This added around $40,000 to our cost estimate, bringing the total to just under $200,000.

It was a lot to ask of the hospital to provide nearly $200,000 of care for free. Fortunately, Brigham had previously worked with the Ray Tye Medical Aid Foundation, a philanthropic organization whose website describes its mission as "funding in-hospital life saving medical treatment and surgeries for those who do not have medical insurance, and for which no other financial resources are available." Their website has countless moving stories of patients from all over the world for whom the foundation has funded surgery in the US. In the upper right corner of the site there is a link for a "Medical Aid Request." I clicked the link, filled out my name, hospital affiliation, and email address; Janel's name, medical condition, and medical needs; a paragraph explaining the team we had assembled at Brigham who would care for him, including specialists in neurology, neurosurgery, oncology, and radiation oncology; and an estimate of the cost of his care at around $200,000. I read it over a few times, then clicked the SUBMIT button.

As a new faculty member, I had a temporary office in a space the Brigham neurology department rented across the street from the hospital, three floors above an ice cream shop. Since the office was tucked away in a location most people didn't even know was part of Brigham, nobody ever dropped in. In fact, scheduling a meeting in the office required giving detailed instructions, and most people got lost trying to find it. The office had no windows, and the fluorescent lights made me lose track of what time of day it was. I didn't spend much time there since I was mostly in the hospital seeing patients or teaching residents and students. But when I was there, it was a quiet refuge from the intense environment of the hospital where I could spend uninterrupted hours focused on the tasks of writing clinic notes, returning patient phone calls, catching up on emails, working on teaching presentations, and trying to write articles.

On the morning after I submitted the online medical aid request form, I was doing just that. It was so quiet and I was so focused on whatever I was working on that I startled when someone knocked on the door.

"Can I transfer a call in to you?" asked one of the call center staff members as I opened the door. The clinic's call center was housed just down the hall from my office.

"Who is it?" I asked anxiously. I was concerned that if someone was knocking rather than just sending an email, it must be some type of patient emergency. Just a few months into practicing independently after nearly a decade of training under the supervision of others, this new level of responsibility still frightened me.

She saw my concern and laughed. "It's not a patient. I think she said she's from a foundation or something?"

Could it be the Ray Tye Medical Aid Foundation? Already?

"Yes, yes, please transfer it," I said. My pulse, already quick from being startled and then worrying about a patient emergency, continued to rise.

The phone rang.

I took a deep breath and focused.

The phone rang again, and I answered. "Hello?"

"Dr. Berkowitz?" a woman's voice asked excitedly, as if she was about to tell me I had won the lottery.

"Yes?" I replied tentatively.

"Oh my Goddddd!" she cried out. "This is Terri from the Ray Tye Medical Aid Foundation. Oh my goodness, we have to help this poor boy!! Can we get him here? Will surgery save him? Tell me how we can get him taken care of here! This is *ex-aaaaac-tly* what we do!"

"Thank you," I managed to stammer out in disbelief. "Thank you so much—"

"I can't wait to meet him!" Terri exclaimed. "We've helped out with soooo many cases from Haiti for PIH. They are amazing! Do you know Dr. Paul Farmer?"

"Well, of course I know of him, but I don't really know him personally . . . I mean, I've read all his books. Well, actually, I guess I shook hands with him after a talk he gave once, but I don't think he'd remember me." I tried to laugh, but it came out as more of a cough. I noticed my hand beginning to cramp from a white-knuckled grip on the phone, and I tried to relax it.

"Paul Farmer is *a-maaaa-zing!*" she nearly sang. "I can't wait to meet this patient! Wait—how do you say his name?"

"It's the French *j*, so more of a *zh* sound: *Zha-nel*," I said.

"When are you going to bring *Zha-nel* here to get his brain tumor out?" she asked.

"Well, to be honest, I didn't expect to have the financial piece solved so quickly." I chuckled nervously. "So we have to see if Brigham will agree and then work on a visa for him."

"I've worked with Brigham many times. They are wonderful! Oh, this poor boy!! Will he be coming with his parents?"

I paused. I had left out the abandonment piece in our aid request letter. Given her excitement, it didn't seem like she was going to change her mind no matter what I told her, and this would have to come out eventually. "Unfortunately, we've learned he was abandoned," I said. "He lives with members of his church—"

"Oh my God, this poor boy," she moaned sincerely. She said she'd talk with the Brigham administration about the costs and logistics. Just as we were about to hang up, I realized I should ask for her email address so we could be in touch—and to make sure I hadn't daydreamed the conversation.

"Well, you're going to laugh," she said, spelling out the address, which concluded @unitedliquors.com. "Mr. Tye made his fortune in the liquor business, working his way up from carrying the cases to running the company."

"Wow," I said, still in shock about the surreal nature of the call.

"So we'll be in touch," she said. "You guys are amazing! PIH, Brigham, all of you do amazing work! And I can't wait to meet Janel!"

"Thank you so much again," I said.

We hung up.

I sat and stared blankly at my computer screen. Was it really this easy—write a letter one day, get $200,000 the next? Slowly my shock and nervous excitement gave way to amazement, to joy, and then finally to curiosity: What was this story of the liquor business?

I Googled "Ray Tye." A World War II veteran, he had risen through the ranks at United Liquors from warehouse worker to president. As his fortune accumulated, he became a philanthropist, stating, "My philosophy is what you take out of this world you put back in." His charitable contributions ranged from paying for individual surgeries of patients in poor and war-torn areas to paying for funerals of local individuals in Boston. "This is not philanthropy. It is a moral responsibility," he was known to say.

Later that day, I received an email that simply said, "Can you help with this?" It was from one of the Brigham administrative leaders, a person I'd never met, though I recognized the name from hospital-wide emails announcing new protocols and policies. Scrolling down, I found a forwarded message sent by the administrators Michelle and I had been speaking with about Janel's case. The email was addressed to all of the hospital's leadership—medical, nursing, social work, care coordination, and executives—and included our free-care request letter and a brief note stating that the Ray Tye Medical Aid Foundation had committed funding. Another member of the administrative leadership team had responded, asking what the plan would be after the patient was discharged from the hospital and whether he would need rehabilitation. It was this set of concerns the person who had emailed me referred to when asking if I could "help with this."

The idea of a young student needing brain surgery tugged on our humanitarian heartstrings. But the hospital administration needed to also consider the perspectives of cost and liability. Thanks to the Ray Tye Medical Aid Foundation, we had solved the cost piece. I presumed the administration's main concern was the possibility of our patient somehow getting stuck in the hospital if there was a prolonged recovery from surgery or a complication causing disability and requiring rehabilitation. Brigham doesn't have an inpatient rehabilitation service, and a recent newspaper article had highlighted the complicated story of a patient who had been brought from Haiti to Boston after the earthquake and was still in a local rehabilitation facility four years later.

I wrote back to the hospital leadership to try to reassure them. I explained that since Janel could walk, presuming the surgery was uncomplicated, there was no reason to believe he wouldn't walk out of the hospital just as he would walk in. In the worst-case scenario, if he required a prolonged postoperative recovery period, I had already

secured a commitment from the rehabilitation center at HUM, and
they were willing and ready to care for him. We could simply fly him
back to Haiti and transport him to HUM. I assured them that if Janel
didn't need rehabilitation but needed to stay in Boston for a few months
of chemotherapy and radiation therapy, we would be able to arrange
local housing for him. Michelle had told me that PIH had coordinated
this many times in the past for other patients who came to the US for
medical care from one of the countries where PIH worked.

The reply from the administrator moments later was one line:

> We really need housing and transport on paper guaranteed
> before.

I hadn't expected the finances to be solved so quickly and easily.
This seemed like a major victory, but we still had a long way to go to
get Janel to Brigham. We needed to figure out housing for him, plus
he would need a visa. Now it seemed that these were linked. To get a
medical visa, we needed Brigham to commit to Janel's care, and to get
Brigham to commit to his care, we needed a plan for housing after he
was discharged from the hospital.

I asked Michelle for ideas the next time I saw her. "Do you and Nina
have an extra room?" she asked, smiling. I couldn't tell if she was jok-
ing. Nina and I had just recently gotten married, and were renting a
small apartment not far from the hospital. We discussed whether we
could have Janel stay with us, but with our work schedules and since we
had only one car between us, we worried we might not be best suited to
take care of him and get him to and from his medical appointments. I
also thought it would be ideal to find someone from the local Haitian
American community to house Janel to at least address the language-
barrier aspect of what was sure to be a difficult period for him. Michelle
sent out emails through her organization to look for volunteers. Nothing came through. It was a lot to ask of someone to house a patient
coming alone from Haiti, undergoing major brain surgery, and staying

in the US for a period of up to two months if he ended up needing chemotherapy and radiation as we suspected he would.

Then Michelle remembered Dr. Anne Beckett. At that time, Anne was an intern in internal medicine and pediatrics, dividing her training between Brigham and Boston Children's Hospital. She had worked for PIH in Haiti for a year during medical school and had been involved in coordinating the care of countless patients sent to the US for surgery after the 2010 earthquake.

Michelle and I called Anne to ask her advice on housing. She explained to us that most of the patients PIH had brought from Haiti to Boston had stayed with Dr. Hermide Mercier. Hermide grew up in Haiti and went to medical school there before moving to Boston in the 1960s, where she studied public health. A leader in the Boston Haitian community, Hermide provided health education through courses and radio and television programs, and worked for the Massachusetts Department of Health on projects related to HIV and tuberculosis. She had also housed nearly two hundred patients for PIH over the preceding decades, including many following the earthquake. PIH called her a "guardian angel."

Anne called Hermide, who said she would be delighted to host Janel. Moreover, several other recovered patients from Haiti who had been living with Hermide since their surgeries were willing to help take care of him. Could it really be that we'd found someone who not only had the time and availability to care for Janel and drive him to appointments but also was a doctor, had help at home, had served in this role countless times, *and* was Haitian? The situation seemed impossibly ideal.

Within a day of contacting Anne, the housing piece had been solved, just as within a day of applying to the Ray Tye Medical Aid Foundation, the financial piece had been solved. It seemed that if we asked the right questions of the right people, we got the answers we were hoping for. With Anne and Hermide offering to join Martineau, Michelle, and me, we felt we had a great team in place to advocate and care for Janel.

Though the negative response from the first neurosurgeons we had contacted had given me pause, the ease and sense of inevitability with which things were beginning to fall into place made it feel like we were on the right track. I felt inspired and humbled to be swept up in PIH's work in this way, and amazed by everyone's generosity toward—and solidarity with—a person they had never even met.

With housing, funding, and a plan for rehabilitation in Haiti (if needed) in place, we got the green light from the Brigham administration to proceed. With evidence of medical necessity and a hospital willing to provide free care, we had what we needed to apply for a visa.

It was early December, three months after Martineau first emailed me about Janel. I was headed back to Haiti.

3

Approaching the departure gate in Miami for my connecting flight, I heard the counterpoint of countless animated Creole conversations, the cacophony of crying babies, and the characteristic chiming of Haitian cell phone ringtones. I smiled. It felt like I was already in Haiti. I sat down and pulled off my overstuffed backpack filled with clothes, a mosquito net, books and neurology journals to catch up on, and a two-week supply of instant oatmeal packets, dehydrated vegetables, ramen noodles, and CLIF bars to supplement the rice-and-beans meals served in the staff house down the road from HUM. I thought about pulling out a neurology journal to leaf through but instead leaned my head against my pack and dozed off. It had been a hectic past few days of packing and taking care of last-minute tasks at work, chores at home, shopping, and phone calls before leaving the country.

Just as I fell asleep, I was jolted awake by people pushing past me and stepping over me. At the first mention of boarding, nearly everyone at the gate made a mad dash for the boarding door. The airport staff tried to direct everyone to look at the boarding group on their tickets. Nobody did. It became clear to the staff that many passengers didn't speak English. A Creole-speaking airport staff member appeared and announced in Creole that passengers should look at the boarding group on their tickets and sit down until their group was called. About half of the passengers looked at their tickets, but most stayed crowded around the entrance to the jet bridge. The gate agents gave up and let everyone board in the order they approached.

Once on the plane, I saw flight attendants resolving conflicts between people who arrived at their assigned seats and the people already sitting in those seats. If your main form of transportation in Haiti is the *taptap*—a pickup truck with a metal roof over the back that fits as many people as can squeeze into it—the idea of an assigned seat may seem foreign. Or even if it's not, if you can't read the ticket, it's hard to figure out your seat assignment. The adult literacy rate in Haiti is only 60 percent, with less than a third of the population going beyond primary school, where most schoolteachers are unqualified or have received minimal training. Even though public school is free, parents must pay for school uniforms and school supplies, costs that are often out of reach.

As I made my way to my seat amid the chaotic boarding process, I passed a wide-eyed flight attendant, her painted-on eyebrows raised nearly to her hairline. "First time flying to Haiti?" I asked.

She nodded slowly, looking past me at the pandemonium.

I smiled at her. "I speak some Creole if you need any help translating," I offered.

She forced a preoccupied smile, then, suddenly alarmed, looked over my head and pushed past me.

"You can't bring that on here, sir!" she shouted to a man trying to fit a large, tattered cardboard box with a television sticking out of it into an overhead bin. He either didn't hear her or didn't understand and kept trying. She tried to approach him and was nearly hit in the head by a huge trash bag of belongings being swung up toward an overhead bin by another passenger, who then tried to stuff it in. I wondered how all of these oversize items had made it through security and how they would fare in cargo when the flight attendants required them to be checked. But can you blame the passengers for trying? I doubt Amazon delivers to rural Haiti.

As we were taxiing to the runway, an elderly man got up from his seat and started walking toward the bathroom. The flight attendants frantically yelled at him (in English) over the intercom system to sit down, but he kept on walking down the aisle. If he could navigate getting into and out of a crowded *taptap* while it swerved on mountainous dirt roads slowing just enough for people to jump on and off, then the enclosed, spacious 737 must have seemed like a safe place to maneuver by comparison, active runway or not. The plane stopped on the runway, and two flight attendants guided the man back to his seat.

Once we made it to cruising altitude, I headed to the bathroom. Opening the door, I nearly bumped into an elderly lady in a broad-brimmed purple church hat who was perched on the toilet with her purple dress pulled up above her waist. I immediately looked away and apologized as I shut the door, but the peeing passenger had seemed completely unfazed. As I turned around, one of the flight attendants sitting behind the bathrooms rolled his eyes and slowly shook his head. "Sorry, they never lock the door on these Haiti flights," he said with disgust before turning back to a solitaire game on his iPad.

Less than a third of Haitians have access to a hygienic latrine, let alone a toilet, so it's common in Haiti to see men, women, and children going to the bathroom along the side of the road. If squatting in plain view of passersby is your standard for privacy, then locking the bathroom door on a plane may seem superfluous, and it might not even bother you if someone accidentally entered. I thought of trying to explain all this to the flight attendant but decided against it. After all, maybe the lady just forgot to lock the door.

For people who have never been to Haiti or airline staff working the route, I worry the chaos that often occurs on these flights reinforces racist stereotypes that have been propagated about Haitians across the ages. From "savages and cannibals" in 1884 to "unthinking black animals" in 1920 (in *National Geographic*); from "illiterate, superstitious, disease-ridden and backward peasants" in the 1970s to "hungry, Satan-worshipping drug addicts . . . branded with the scarlet H [of HIV]" in the 1980s and 1990s. Haiti was referred to as a "black hole" by *Vanity*

Fair in 1989 and a "shithole" by Donald Trump in 2018. When we are primed by such stereotypes, we are prone to reinforce them—we may notice and remember what fulfills our preexisting beliefs rather than realize, for example, that most people on a flight to Haiti are following all of the normal procedures just like us.

Increasingly, all flights to Haiti have either a Creole-speaking flight attendant or an additional Creole-speaking staff member there just to translate. On one flight, I heard a Creole-speaking crew member amend the usual safety information announcement to address nearly all of the unexpected things I'd seen regularly on flights to and from Haiti. When she mentioned an infant changing table being available in the bathroom, she added, "So please don't change your baby in your seat." When she said the bit about not tampering with bathroom smoke detectors, she added, "When you're in the bathroom, please lock the door," and she explained how. She also noted, "In the bathroom you will see a blue button that says 'flush.' Please press this after you go so the next person doesn't see what you did." After finishing with the formalities of what to do in the unlikely event of a water landing or a loss of cabin pressure, she stated, "If you brought something that doesn't fit below your seat or above—like a television— please tell us so we can check it. If you don't know how to read your ticket, ask us so we can show you to your seat. You can't walk around while the plane is moving on the ground, taking off, or landing. If you do this, we won't be able to get you where you're trying to go." She concluded, "Now it's time to turn off your phones. Say goodbye to your son or daughter, tell them to send you five thousand dollars, and hang up." The passengers erupted in laughter.

I wondered if the other flight attendants had any idea that she had tailored the standard safety script to try to avoid some of the common mishaps and misunderstandings on these flights. And I wondered if they realized that each element of what must seem so "backward" to them has an important explanation rooted in Haiti's dire poverty and the historical forces that gave rise to it.

Another striking aspect of flights to and from Haiti is the line of a dozen or more wheelchair-bound passengers waiting to board. I initially presumed this was a depressing reflection of the number of disabled patients in Haiti due to lack of access to healthcare and the more than one million people injured in the 2010 earthquake. But the more I traveled to Haiti, the more I noticed that among the elderly and infirm passengers who clearly needed wheelchairs, some wheelchair passengers looked quite well, and quite well-to-do. Once I thought I even saw someone who had boarded in a wheelchair later walking around on the flight, but I wasn't sure it was the same person. Could it be that some passengers were using wheelchairs as a sort of VIP experience to be carted around at the airport and board first? I felt bad for even thinking this. But Haiti does have its elite, the less than 0.1 percent who hold all the wealth and live lives of luxury while most of the population struggles to survive.

The privileged are not hard to spot on these flights. Once I saw two very well-dressed light-skinned Haitian women become upset when they discovered their seats were in the last row in front of the restrooms. They called the flight attendant over and explained in perfect, barely accented English that they absolutely could not sit in the back of the plane.

The flight attendant looked at their tickets. "But that's where your assigned seats are, ladies," she explained kindly.

"You can't make us sit near the bathroom!" one of the women scolded her.

"No, no! Absolutely not!" the other chimed in. "We have allergies! So we most certainly can*not*!"

"Yes, very *bad* allergies!" the first woman concurred, nodding vigorously. They stood with their arms crossed, refusing to sit in their assigned seats.

The flight attendant looked at them quizzically and then shrugged. She said she would see if there were empty seats in another part of the plane.

These ladies reminded me of the rare wealthy patients we see in our neurology clinic at HUM who come because they have heard a foreign neurologist was visiting. They always try to be seen first without going through the normal registration process, which we of course politely refuse. Rather than the usual neurologic complaints of our local patients—headache, seizures, paralysis—these wealthy patients almost never actually have anything wrong with them, at least nothing neurological. They nearly always complain of nothing more than a vague malaise, which we had come to jokingly call "Petionvillitis," since it seemed to be described only by healthy and wealthy people from the rich Port-au-Prince suburb of Petionville. I had never been there, but colleagues told me it was like stepping outside Haiti: fancy restaurants, luxurious hotels, and government officials dressed like movie stars eating dinner with security details surrounding them. Though we reassure our Petionvillitis patients that with a normal neurological examination it was very unlikely they had any underlying neurologic condition, they often try to convince us to do CT scans of their brains "just to make sure." Even after we kindly refuse, they tend to linger in the clinic, seemingly just to chat, until my colleagues and I insist we need to see our other patients.

These rare wealthy visitors to our clinic conduct themselves so differently from the rest of our patients, who often patiently wait all day to be seen, sometimes even sleeping the night before outside the hospital on a blanket, a folded cardboard box, or nothing at all to ensure they will be seen early enough on the day of their appointment to make it home before nightfall, or before the late-afternoon rains make the river they have to cross to get home too high to safely traverse.

On one flight, I was traveling with a Haitian colleague from Mirebalais, and I decided to ask her about my wheelchair theory. "I've noticed that there are so many people in wheelchairs on these flights. Some are clearly quite elderly or look sick, but others, they look okay. I don't want to judge, but do you think some people could just be using them as a sort of VIP chariot?"

She laughed. "Let's study it," she proposed, smiling.

She had just undergone surgery herself, and so we boarded early in the needing-more-time-down-the-jet-bridge group just behind the wheelchair passengers. Sure enough, as we approached the door to the plane, we saw one well-dressed woman dexterously shimmy out of her wheelchair, step over the footrests, and walk confidently onto the plane—in high heels!

My colleague looked at me with a surprised smile. "Maybe your hypothesis is correct!" she whispered, trying not to laugh.

Another gentleman we had noted in the wheelchair line looked young and healthy. He was dressed in a neatly pressed white suit. I tried to give him the benefit of the doubt. Perhaps he had been in an accident or had some type of childhood-onset illness that had left him paralyzed but he was otherwise well. We later saw him walking up and down the aisle talking to friends throughout the flight and easily navigating the chaotic baggage claim area in Port-au-Prince.

From illiteracy to entitlement and corruption, from going to the bathroom with the door open to refusing to sit near the bathroom, Haiti's inequities and their juxtaposition are in plain view before even arriving there.

I fell asleep soon after we were in the air, exhausted from having taken a 6 a.m. flight from Boston to make the Port-au-Prince connection in Miami that would arrive early enough in the afternoon for me to get to Mirebalais before dark. When I woke up, I looked out the window to see the sparkling blue Caribbean Sea turn turquoise as it made contact with Haiti's coastline. A beautiful, pristine beach. But there were no resorts, no hotels. The land was a mix of barren browns and bleached-out whites, colorless compared to the rich blue hue of the ocean. Small winding dirt roads snaked over treeless mountains sprinkled with sparse specks that blindingly reflected the midday sunlight—tin roofs of houses in groups of no more than a dozen, nothing that could even be called a village.

The passenger in the seat behind me made a few clicking *tsk-tsk* sounds. *"Gade, peyi nou vid!"* he said with a twinge of disgust. ("Look, our country is *empty!*")

This northwest corner of Haiti wasn't always empty. When Columbus landed at this exact location on his famous 1492 voyage, he described an island coast "full of trees of a thousand kinds . . . wonderful pine-groves and very large plains of verdure . . . so beautiful and rich" with "a population of incalculable number," whom he admired as intelligent, kind, attractive, and generous, "as though they would give their hearts." Indeed the native Taíno people would give their hearts and more. In spite of Columbus's praise for the Taíno, he enslaved them to farm and mine their land. Slavery and associated starvation, slaughter, and suicide—along with susceptibility to smallpox and other imported European diseases—led to the extinction of the Taíno in less than a century. The Old World's first New World genocide complete, the Spanish conquistadors moved on to Central and South America. So began the emptying of Haiti.

France subsequently took control of the territory and imported hundreds of thousands of slaves from West Africa. Though the French refilled the island with people, they began emptying it of its natural resources—after depositing the slaves, they sent the emptied slave ships back to Europe filled with timber from trees felled to make way for sugar plantations, beginning Haiti's deforestation.

On the backs of the slaves, the French created a colony so rich from sugar and coffee exports that at its peak it generated more revenue than the thirteen North American colonies combined. Atrocious and often deadly conditions for slaves led to revolts, which exploded into full-blown revolution. So valuable was the colony to France that Napoleon sent his naval fleet to attempt to maintain control of it. But the rebel slaves were victorious, defeating Napoleon's forces in history's only successful slave uprising. Haiti became the second European colony to declare independence after the US.

The US refused to acknowledge its newly independent neighbor out of fear of the implications for its own slaves—US slavery would persist for sixty years following Haitian independence. France also shunned its former colony, offering diplomatic recognition only after Haiti grudgingly agreed to pay France an indemnity for loss of property— property that included the former slaves themselves. Another historical first and last—a war's victor paying the defeated nation for its losses—payments on the indemnity (estimated at three billion dollars in modern currency) continued for over a century, often under threat of force. Emptied of its native people, emptied of its natural resources, Haiti suffered the emptying of its coffers.

The ensuing devastating poverty led to continuous tumult marked by coups, corruption, assassinations, a twenty-year US military occupation, and a thirty-year father-son totalitarian dictatorship. Haiti would wait nearly two hundred years from its founding to have its first peaceful transfer of power from a democratically elected leader who had served a full term to another democratically elected leader. The fourteen years preceding this milestone saw thirteen transfers of power.

Zealous slave importation by the French had left Haiti with a population seven times higher than that of the neighboring Dominican Republic despite being half its size. Overpopulation required more land to farm and more fuel with which to cook, leading to further deforestation to clear the land and to make charcoal. The loss of what few trees remained made the soil less fertile and more prone to erosion and landslides when hurricanes battered Haiti's shores. As farming failed, rural peasants migrated in droves to Port-au-Prince to seek low-wage factory jobs, overcrowding the capital with urban slums, which set the stage for the toll of death, disability, displacement, and destruction from the 2010 earthquake to be orders of magnitude higher than that from any other earthquake of the same force elsewhere.

And so this once verdant and populous northwest region beneath our plane's path became empty—deforested first by French greed, then by Haitian necessity; depopulated first by genocide of the Taíno, then centuries later by mass migration from the countryside to the city due to deforestation and destitute poverty.

"Gade, peyi nou vid," the passenger behind me said again, somberly this time. ("Look, our country is empty.")

His neighbor joined in the lament: *"E si ou malad la, kote ou prale?"* ("And if you got sick out there, where would you go?")

———————

I made my way through the chaotic, stuffy baggage claim area to the exit of the Port-au-Prince airport. In the small exit hallway, I bought minutes for my Haitian cell phone (a small pre-flip era model) and called my local PIH contact to see if the driver was there before I ventured out of the airport into what's referred to as the "VIP parking lot," a fenced-in lot jam-packed with cars pointing every which way.

The first few times I came to Haiti, I found exiting the airport nerve-wracking and a little scary. Would the ride PIH was supposed to set up actually be there? Would I recognize the driver? Could I be led astray by someone pretending to be my driver wanting to rob or kidnap me? Nothing like this has ever happened in Haiti to me or anyone I know, but the US Department of State Travel Advisory for Haiti reads:

*Reconsider Travel to Haiti due to **crime, civil unrest, and kidnapping**.*

> *Protests, tire burning, and road blockages are frequent and unpredictable. Violent crime, such as armed robbery, is common, and incidents of kidnapping have occurred. Local police may lack the resources to respond effectively to serious criminal incidents, and emergency response, including ambulance service, is limited or nonexistent. Travelers are sometimes targeted, followed, and violently attacked and robbed shortly after leaving the Port-au-Prince international airport.*

As I exited the airport into the crowd of people awaiting arriving passengers and taxi drivers eager to offer me a ride, I remembered my first trip to Haiti. There had been no phone contact. I had been told someone would meet me at the airport exit, but of the hundreds of people waiting there, nobody had clearly appeared to be waiting for me. I had wandered through the parking lot trying to look as if I knew where I was going, though I had no idea. To my relief, I had eventually found my ride: an ambulance from the hospital where I would be working. I had looked on a map and seen the hospital was about eighty miles west of the airport, so I had estimated a two-hour trip. After we had navigated the narrow, hilly city streets of Port-au-Prince and got out onto a coastal highway, that seemed to be a reasonable estimate. Then we had taken a hard left off the coastal highway and into the forest, bouncing and bumping along dirt roads (were they even roads? It got dark and I couldn't tell) and then through a river, the headlights illuminating the muddy water in the darkness like some odd submarine. We had arrived at the hospital four and a half hours later.

This time, just after I passed through an opening in the chain-link fence of the parking lot, a PIH driver emerged from the crowd and waved me over. As we squeezed between bumpers of tightly packed rows of cars, he asked me how I was and how my family was, and I did the same. We got into the white PIH van, and he cranked up the air-conditioning and the *kompa*, a Haitian musical genre aptly described by one journalist as the "thumping love child of merengue, funk, and R&B." As we maneuvered out of the parking lot, I noticed I was nodding my head in time with the groovy beat and funky synthesizer riffs. I smiled. It was good to be back in Haiti. I counted that it was my fourth trip, and I felt like I was starting to get the hang of things.

The driver weaved jerkily through narrow city streets pockmarked with potholes. He shifted gears frequently, honking at every near miss with a person, car, motorcycle, stray dog, goat, or one of the ubiquitous *taptaps*. Brightly painted in a combination of red, yellow, blue, and orange, these pickup-truck taxis ply the roads all over Haiti, picking up and dropping off passengers who squeeze into the back by the dozens. *Taptaps* have names painted across the tops of their windshields, some in French, some in Creole, some in English. Most names are religious. There are those that address God (*L'homme propose, Dieu dispose* [Man proposes, God provides]; *Dye seul protej* [Only God protects]; *Dieu sait tout* [God knows all]; *Dye w fidel* [God you are faithful]; *Bondye beni w* [God bless you]; *Je crois en Dieu* [I believe in God]; *Grace de Dieu* [Grace of God]; God is good; In God we trust) and those that address Jesus (*Merci, Jesus* [Thank you, Jesus]; *Gloire à Jesus* [Glory to Jesus]; *Jezi prezan* [Jesus is present]; *Christ revient* [Christ returns]; *Christ capable* [Christ is capable]) and those that make biblical references (*Sélon Jean* [According to John]; Mt. Carmel; Ebenezer; *Grace divine* [Divine Grace]) and those that simply cite a biblical chapter and verse, the most popular being Psalm 23:1 (The Lord is my shepherd, I lack nothing), Psalm 34:8 (Taste and see that the Lord is good; blessed is the one who takes refuge in him), and Exodus 14:14 (The Lord will fight for you; you need only to be still). Some express a state of mind (*Nostalgie*, *La perseverance, Patience, La Deliverance*), while others state a credo (Never die, One love, First class). *Taptaps* are painted with everything from religious images to the Batman symbol to the New York Yankees logo to the faces of basketball players from the NBA to suggestively dressed women with exaggerated proportions.

After bumpy stop-and-go maneuvering through the crowded streets of Port-au-Prince, the driver floored it on a brief straight stretch of highway that led toward the mountains. But once we reached the mountains, he slowed to navigate the steep and winding ascent, passing frighteningly close to perilous drop-offs while dump trucks overloaded with huge rocks traveled down in the opposite direction looking like they were about to topple over, and motorcycles carrying whole families of unhelmeted passengers coasted down past them with their engines off to save gas.

After forty-five vertiginous minutes on the mountain roads, we crossed a small bridge over a muddy river where women were washing clothes, kids were splashing around, and trash of all kinds lined the banks. The car bumped along on a chalky white dirt road past tin-roofed shacks and small wooden market stalls, the streets bustling with people and motorcycles. Suddenly a gleaming, single-story white building adorned with shield-size medallions of intricate local iron-worker art came into view: Hôpital Universitaire de Mirebalais—HUM—the largest solar-powered hospital in a low-income country anywhere in the world.

HUM looks like it fell out of the sky. The sharp angles of the hospital's white walls topped with rows of glistening solar panels contrast with the gently sloping green hills behind it. Stray dogs and chickens graze out front on the tree-lined cobblestone path to the entrance. Just across the street from the hospital, pigs rummage through a trash-filled gutter that lines a dirt road leading into a village of one-room shacks, some wooden, some concrete, most with no electricity or running water. The village is roamed by cows, donkeys, mules, and roosters outdoors, and by rats, geckos, mosquitos, and tarantulas indoors.

The longer I face the complexities and challenges of working in Haiti, the more of a marvel HUM seems. The earthquake that devastated Haiti occurred in 2010, and HUM, part of the reconstruction effort, opened in 2013. A hospital requires not only the structure itself but also, as Paul Farmer likes to say, "space, staff, stuff, and systems." PIH and its Haitian sister organization, Zanmi Lasante—which means Partners In Health in Haitian Creole and goes by ZL for short—somehow managed to conceive of, plan, build, and staff a hospital of this magnitude in this place in less than three years. And they didn't just open a fully staffed hospital; they launched postgraduate medical training programs in internal medicine, surgery, pediatrics, and obstetrics-gynecology—the first such programs outside a major city in Haiti.

How did PIH and ZL take this project from idea to realization so fast?

It seemed impossible: from buying the plot of land through a complex and often dysfunctional governmental bureaucracy to commissioning architectural plans to hiring staff, from security guards to surgeons, secretaries to seasoned hospital administrators. Paul Farmer often says that the only failures are failures of imagination. I have an image in my mind of PIH's strategy as throwing a ball from one end of a football field and then running as quickly as possible to catch it at the other end. Somehow the strategy worked. HUM is a testament to the depth and breadth of PIH/ZL's thirty-year commitment to and collaboration with the communities they serve, their experience building health systems in some of the world's poorest communities, and the visionary imagination of their leadership.

We turned onto a smaller dirt road and then a smaller one. We stopped abruptly in front of a red metal gate with barbed wire along the top. The driver beeped twice. He beeped twice again. Slowly, the red gate started moving, pulled open by a security guard. The driver shifted into gear, and the van lurched through the gate. We had arrived at the HUM staff house, a two-floor concrete building with eight bedrooms, two bathrooms, a kitchen, and a dining room.

Opening the car door and stepping out from the comfortable air-conditioning, I was assaulted by the sweltering temperature and heavy humidity. One of the local women who works in the house came out to greet me, kissing me on each sweaty cheek. She asked how my wife was and whether we had children yet. I told her we didn't. "Not yet!" she said and laughed. She led me upstairs to the room I would be staying in for two weeks. My back soaked with sweat under my backpack as we climbed the stairs to the second floor, where it felt 10 degrees warmer than the first floor. She opened the wooden door to a small room, and dense heat seemed to explode out of it. She flicked on the ceiling light, a plain fixture filled with dead bugs that had flown into the heat of its bulb and died. The room was just barely able to fit a wooden twin bed with a faded peach-colored sheet on it, a wooden desk with a metal folding chair, a small wooden armoire, and a white circulating fan, which she plugged in and turned on. I dropped off my backpack and headed back downstairs.

I ate some rice and beans left over from lunch and then took a refreshing cold shower under a trickling rusted showerhead. But as soon as I dried off, I could already feel droplets of sweat beginning to emerge from every pore. After returning to my room, I set up my mosquito net over the bed, crawled under it with a neurology journal, and pulled the small fan next to my flushed, overheated face. The circulating hot air felt more like a blow-dryer than a fan but provided some small relief. I tried to read but fell asleep with the lights on, exhausted from the day of travel and my abrupt transition from Boston's winter to Haiti's oppressive tropical heat.

4

t was only 7:30 a.m. and the temperature was already in the high 80s. Walking from the staff house to HUM, I traversed an open dirt area that local kids use as a soccer field, the goals made of two tree branches stuck into holes in the ground with a strand of twine running between them. There was no one playing soccer this early in the morning. Instead, a few emaciated mules, cows, and goats grazed, tethered to wooden posts in the ground. I crossed the field to the chalky, rocky dirt road that leads to the hospital. People stood in front of their one-room wooden and concrete tin-roofed houses in their underwear, scrubbing themselves with soapy water from buckets—morning baths in a place with no plumbing.

My Haitian colleagues and I had decided to try a new model for this visit. On previous trips, I'd given lectures on neurology topics to the entire staff of HUM and seen patients with any doctor who asked for a neurologic consultation. I had tried to make each consultation educational for whoever wanted my help, but this strategy had led to me teaching a little bit to a lot of people rather than teaching a lot to a few people who could master the information. On this trip, we had decided I would work with only Martineau and a group of five HUM internal medicine residents, and they would work with only me. Martineau invited all of his most challenging neurologic patients to come for a consultation and encouraged his colleagues from all of the other departments at HUM—internal medicine, pediatrics, surgery, mental health—to save up their neurology consults for this week so we could see a large number of patients together.

As I crossed the street separating the village from the hospital, the smell of various meats simmering in spices mingled with the cloud of diesel and dust from the road. The cobblestone area in front of the entrance to HUM was bustling with women selling various items to patients and their families. Some sat behind wicker baskets of neatly arranged hard-boiled eggs, bunches of bananas, or plastic pouches of popcorn. Others sold sodas, juices, and small plastic sachets of purified water out of ice-filled coolers balanced on rusted wheelbarrows. And some vendors opened metal containers to reveal steaming mixtures of rice, beans, goat, and chicken. Scrawny stray dogs panted patiently nearby, hoping for a scrap. Men walked motorcycles around, looking for customers in search of a ride home.

PIH recognized early on that health is not only about medicine but also about combating poverty. Beyond all of the local jobs created by the hospital itself, the informal economy outside HUM thrives, providing provisions for waiting patients, their family members, and hospital staff as well as a source of income for the community.

I passed through the improvised market to the hospital entrance, marked by the PIH logo of four cartoon-like hands reaching toward each other from the four sides of a square. I imagined this symbolized the Haitian proverb *Men anpil chay pa lou* (Many hands make the burden lighter). Just inside the entrance, a crowd of patients swarmed around the registration desk, reminding me of the boarding process for my flight the prior morning. Having a hospital of this capacity where there was none previously opened the floodgates—more than a thousand patients pass through HUM every day.

I weaved through the crowd to get to Martineau's clinic room and found him seated at his desk.

"Doc Aaron!" he said, standing, smiling, and slapping his hand into mine for a firm handshake. He leaned down to hug me with the other arm.

"Doc Martineau!" I said, hugging him back. Martineau is just a few years younger than I am. Tall and slender, he wears slim-fitting button-down shirts and slacks that make him look even taller and more slender. He has almond-shaped eyes and keeps his hair cropped close but his goatee full.

"How was the trip?" he asked with just the slightest hint of a Haitian accent, smiling broadly.

"Good! Happy to be back," I said, returning his smile. "Do you have a lot of patients coming for us this week?"

"A lot of patients!" he said enthusiastically, still smiling. "A lot of very difficult patients! I hope you can help me with them."

"I'll try," I said.

"And one patient is coming today who I know you are going to be very interested to see," he said, nodding slowly, his smile gradually fading. "You will get to meet Janel today."

"Wow," I said. I was excited to finally meet this patient who had occupied my thoughts, my emails, and my conversations for the last three months. I'd seen pictures of his brain and a video of his reflexes, but I hadn't seen *him*. I imagined he would be excited too, finally meeting the doctor who had been advocating for him to get his surgery for free in the US.

Martineau had indeed made sure we'd see a lot of patients. Crammed into the small clinic room, sitting on the desk, examination table, and chairs, he and I, along with the five residents, made new diagnoses of Parkinson's disease, epilepsy, and migraine that morning alone. Fortunately these are all conditions that we could treat with medications available in Haiti. But we also saw patients with odd constellations of neurologic symptoms and signs, who remained diagnostic mysteries. We hoped a CT scan might help us with at least some of them.

Later in the day, one of the residents picked up a patient chart from the stack of tan folders on the clinic room's desk and opened the door. "Janel!" she shouted into the waiting room, where a crowd of hundreds of patients sat on wooden benches, with hundreds more standing around them.

I stood and went to the doorway, looking around expectantly for a young college-age man to emerge from the crowd. My pulse quickened. Would we shake hands or would we hug? Would he be scared of his upcoming trip to the US? Or would he be excited to go to *lòt bò a*—the other side—in spite of the circumstances?

"Janel!" the resident shouted again, louder, trying to be heard above the din of conversations, crying babies, and ringing cell phones.

A corner of the crowd parted, revealing a thin elderly woman pushing a wheelchair with a young man in it. He was wide-eyed, staring forward. His nose was broad and dignified, offset by a short, thin mustache just above his upper lip. His hair was cropped close. He wore a tan suit, white button-down shirt, and dark blue tie—patients often come to the hospital in their Sunday best.

The elderly woman pushed the wheelchair through the doorway, stepped away from it, and leaned against a wall in the corner of the crowded clinic room. The young man sat silently.

Why is he in a wheelchair? I wondered. I had imagined he would walk in.

The residents looked at him, at each other, and then back at him.

I tried greeting him in Creole and asking how he was. He stared at me with eyes that seemed to bulge, blinking slowly and infrequently. He didn't respond. Maybe it was my Creole. Martineau asked him how he was—was he doing well? After a long pause, Janel croaked out a high-pitched, raspy *"Wi"* ("Yes"), barely parting his lips to make the sound.

We examined him. Looking at his eyes, I realized that his wide-eyed stare was a result of retraction of his eyelids and because he had difficulty looking upward, elements of what is called Parinaud's syndrome—a condition I'd read about but hadn't seen before. Parinaud's syndrome is caused by pathology of the dorsal midbrain, a structure at the base of the brain where the centers that control the eyelids and vertical gaze reside. Part of Janel's tumor was pressing on this region.

When we asked Janel to lift his arms and legs, he did this slowly, barely moving. His right hand trembled rapidly as I'd seen in the video Martineau had sent me months prior. We wanted to evaluate his walking, but he was too unsteady on his feet. When Martineau and I tried to help Janel up by his arms, he wobbled and collapsed back into the wheelchair.

I was confused, trying to reconcile the image of the patient I'd formed in my mind with the person in front of me. How could this wheelchair-bound young man who was barely able to move or speak still be going to college?

"Is he worse?" I asked Martineau anxiously.

"*Leggierement,*" he said matter-of-factly. ("Slightly.")

"I thought . . ." I started and trailed off. "I thought you said he was a student?" I asked.

"He was, but he had to stop going to school," Martineau said. He exchanged a few phrases in Creole with the lady in the corner who had brought Janel. I couldn't follow what they were saying. "He made it to fourth grade," Martineau translated for me.

"Fourth grade at twenty-three years old?" I asked, surprised.

Martineau nodded slowly, unfazed.

"And who is the woman with him?" I asked.

"That's his mom," Martineau said.

"His mom?" I asked, my eyebrows rising. "I thought you said he'd been abandoned?"

"Yes, that was the original story we heard," he said. "But it turns out his mom could not take care of him anymore so Janel went to live with a man at their church. But she is still involved. She visits him there and helps take care of him."

My thoughts were racing. We had been advocating in Boston to the hospital and donors for a college student who'd been abandoned by his family who wouldn't need any rehabilitation after surgery. Our exact words had been that we expected he would "walk into the hospital" and then "walk back out." It turned out that none of this was true. Sure, stories evolve as new details emerge, like the story of abandonment. But the rest had likely been my own imagination.

When I saw "twenty-three-year-old student" in Martineau's initial email, I had assumed college. But due to the poverty in Haiti that causes children to start school late and have frequent interruptions, many older students are still in early grades. In Janel's case, perhaps the tumor had been growing for a long time, causing him to have difficulty thinking, remembering, and paying attention, which had impaired his progress in school. With his minimal ability to interact and move, it was hard to even imagine how he would participate in fourth grade.

When I saw the video of Janel on the examination table, I had presumed he'd climbed up there on his own. In reality, he must have been lifted onto it. Of course, if he could walk and talk, why would he have been abandoned? It appeared obvious in retrospect. I had formed a strong but completely inaccurate impression based on the image I had constructed in my mind of an otherwise healthy twenty-three-year-old student from reading into the email, watching the video, and my desire to see—and make—a big save. Suddenly it seemed I had gravely misinterpreted everything.

How would all of this have played out if we had known from the beginning that Janel was barely able to talk or move? Ian, the neurosurgeon, might have thought Janel's condition was too advanced to undergo surgery. The hospital administrators might have been reluctant to commit to his case, given the risks of brain surgery at his level of disability and the level of care he'd need before and after his operation. Hermide, the generous woman who had agreed to house Janel, might have been less willing to do so if she had known he was so disabled that his own mother couldn't care for him. And, sadly, the hospital and donors supporting Janel's care might have found the story of a bedbound twenty-three-year-old fourth grade student less compelling than the sensational story of a college student whose studies were cut short by a progressive but curable tumor and who had no family to support him.

I even had to ask myself whether I would have gone through all of the work and advocacy of the preceding three months if I had known how bad off Janel was. Of course he still would have been a young man suffering from a disease potentially treatable in the US. But with the disease process so advanced, would I have thought of him in the same big-save sort of way? Or would I have felt that he was just too far down the path of his disease for it to make sense to mobilize all of the resources needed to get him to Boston for a high-risk surgery? I wasn't sure.

So what was I supposed to do? Should I just keep moving forward since we had come this far? Even if it was probably too late to expect surgery would make him better, maybe it could at least prevent him from getting worse. Or had the first neurosurgeons been right after all, that a palliative approach made sense given the severity of his condition? Should I go back to everyone in Boston, sheepishly apologize for unintentionally misinforming them, and see how they responded? If I shifted course at this point, it would make me look naïve and unprofessional for taking things this far without really knowing the full story. It could even jeopardize my chance of ever bringing another patient from Haiti to Boston in the future, even a more straightforward case with a better chance of being a big save.

And what about asking Janel what he wanted? Martineau had said he'd discussed everything with him, but Janel didn't look like he could eke out more than one-word answers. Did he really understand what was happening? Even if he did, how could he communicate that he understood?

I tried not to let my distress show.

"Are you ready to come to Boston?" I tried to ask Janel in my still-novice Creole.

He stared at me, expressionless, blinking slowly.

Martineau translated, asking him in more grammatically correct Creole.

After a few moments he croaked out another *"Wi"* ("Yes") in his pinched, high-pitched voice.

"It's going to be cold," I said, mimicking a shiver and smiling nervously.

He continued to stare at me.

Again, Martineau translated my clunky attempt into grammatically correct Creole, chuckling.

No response.

Martineau gave me a brisk nod. We were falling behind, and it was time to move on to the next patient.

"Oke, n'a we Boston," I said to Janel, putting out my hand to shake. ("Okay, we'll see each other in Boston.")

He stared at me. Then he slowly lifted his right hand a few inches off his lap. It quivered with a fine tremor and then began to shake more wildly. He put it back down on his thigh. The shaking stopped.

His mom wheeled him out, and they disappeared into the sea of people in the waiting area. How would she get him home? They had borrowed one of the hospital's wheelchairs, she was thin and elderly, and Janel was too big to be carried. Somehow she'd gotten him to HUM. She must have found help along the way to hoist him up onto a *taptap* or motorcycle.

Martineau and the residents called the next patient in and began their evaluation, and I slipped out to find Michelle, who happened to be at HUM that same week. I had texted her to come see Janel with me, but she was in a meeting and said to check in with her afterward.

"How was it?" she asked, smiling excitedly.

I closed my eyes and frowned, shaking my head.

"What's wrong?" she asked.

"He looks terrible," I said. "He can't talk, and he can't even stand, let alone walk."

"So he really needs that surgery!" she said, squinting seriously at me and nodding firmly, setting her large, dangling, teardrop-shaped silver earrings into perpetual motion.

"And he wasn't abandoned," I groaned. "His mom came in with him."

She laughed. "Stories often change here."

"But I feel like we sold a completely false story to the hospital and the donors," I said.

"It's not a false story. It's the best information we had at the time," she said nonchalantly.

"But he's not even a college student, he's a fourth grade student," I said. "*Was* a fourth grade student," I corrected myself. "He's no longer in school."

"Do you think he can still benefit from surgery?" she asked, making it clear by her tone that she already had the answer in mind.

"Well, clearly he will only get worse without it . . ." I began.

"So then we're on the right track!" She smiled again. "Just tell everyone he's gotten worse, which is true. I have to run to another meeting. Keep me posted!" She dashed off.

I stood alone for a moment, confused. Then I went back to the clinic to keep working with the residents and Martineau.

That night I called Anne, our colleague in Boston who had connected us with Hermide and had extensive experience bringing patients from Haiti to Boston. I updated her about how Janel was not the twenty-three-year-old college student I had imagined—he was severely neurologically impaired. I told her how I couldn't help but wonder if we would have gone through all of the trouble to try to get Janel to Boston if we had known how bad off he was from the beginning. I explained to her how I was worried about momentum carrying us forward since we'd worked so hard to advocate for him to get surgery in the US, but I felt we needed to pause and reconsider our plans given the shifting landscape. I was eager for her advice and perspective.

"Well, I'm not sure if I ever told you, but my brother has Down's syndrome," she said. "If he developed a brain tumor, we'd definitely want him to have surgery if it could help him."

I immediately felt awful. I had prided myself on aspiring to embody PIH's principle to value all lives equally and advocate for access to the best healthcare for the poorest patients. And yet in my questioning of what we were doing, I had fallen short of living up to this ideal. This young man was suffering. His mom was suffering watching her son suffer. We had the chance to help him. Why should his current condition affect his chances of getting a surgery that might be able to improve or at least extend his life?

I apologized to Anne for being insensitive, but if I'd offended her she didn't let on. She calmly assured me that Hermide could care for Janel even if he was bedbound, as she had taken care of countless patients with varying degrees of disability. I tried to clear my head of any doubt about moving forward with bringing him to the US for surgery.

But I still wondered how much Janel understood about what was going on. I regretted that I hadn't tried to talk with his mother, but I had been too preoccupied by how sick Janel looked to even think of it. The next day I asked Martineau if we could call her together.

"She doesn't have a phone," he said. He smiled at my naïve surprise that we had no way to reach her. "They are really poor," he explained. "But you can call Wilner. He's the man from Janel's church who has been taking care of him in his home. He says he speaks for Janel and his family. I'm not sure why he didn't come yesterday. He probably had to work."

I called Wilner and introduced myself. I explained that we had gotten free surgery for Janel approved in the US, but I wanted to make sure that he and Janel's family understood the potential outcomes: Janel could get better, he could stay the same, or he could get worse. He could even die.

"We understand," Wilner said calmly. "After all, this is true of any medical intervention, is it not, Doctor?"

He was, of course, right. I could tell from how he spoke—and the fact that we could communicate in French rather than Creole—that he was far more educated than anyone in Janel's family. Janel's fourth grade education was likely more than his parents would have had. Maybe Wilner was entrusted to speak for them because they respected him as an educated member of their church. He assured me that Janel and his family would be willing to take whatever risk necessary to try to improve his condition.

The rest of my trip was jam-packed with patient consults and teaching. I enjoyed watching Martineau and the medical residents progress in neurology, applying what they learned from one patient to the next. But each night when I left the hospital and lay down under my mosquito net, my mind spun in time with the fan as it blew hot air against my face. Had I inadvertently misled everyone about Janel's situation based on my misinterpretation of Martineau's original email? If so, would they now reconsider their offers when we told them? And should *I* reconsider whether we should keep moving forward given how much worse off Janel was than we had expected? But even if he was in such bad shape, why should he deserve less than the person we had imagined him to be? And then there was still the issue of whether he and his family truly understood the risks and potential benefits of surgery since we'd not been able to ask them directly.

On the last day of my trip, I went to talk to Père (Father) Eddy about the situation. A priest, psychologist, and director of PIH/ZL's mental health program in Haiti, Père Eddy had become one of my closest colleagues there. He had been a great mentor to me over the preceding years, teaching me a lot about Haitian culture, and doing so with a mix of compassionate warmth and razor-sharp wit.

I told him the story up to that point. "I'm worried about whether the patient really understands the risks of this surgery," I said. "If he really does, maybe he would choose to stay home with his family and let nature take its course." I thought about how Haitians often accompany expressions as mundane as "See you tomorrow" with the qualifier *si Bondye vle* ("if God wants").

"If there is any chance he can be helped, no matter what the risk may be, he will want this," Père Eddy began calmly, holding my gaze with his. "His family will want this. His community will want this. His doctors here will want this." He had built to a bit of a crescendo. Then he said more softly, "You have not misunderstood that."

I nodded, listening to him intently.

"Your misunderstanding comes from your conception of patient autonomy!" he said rapidly, and then smiled broadly. "Where you come from, you give the patient the *choice*. Here, doctors tell patients what *needs* to be *done*. Or they just do it. Patients don't want you to *ask* them what they *want*; they want you to *tell* them what they *need*! Based on *your* assessment of the risks and benefits, not theirs. You understand?"

Were my attempts to be sensitive to the situation turning out to be insensitive? Père Eddy seemed to suggest that I was misapplying my homegrown ethics in this foreign context.

"You always help me translate what's happening here," I said, feeling a little relief. "Thank you."

"Haiti is a complex land!" he said and laughed. "Here's another proverb for your collection." He knew I loved learning Haitian proverbs. *"Tout sa ou we se pa sa."*

I smiled, liking the sound of it, but I hadn't understood it. "One more time?" I asked him.

He said it again, more slowly. *"Tout . . . sa . . . ou . . . we . . . se . . . pa . . . sa."* He smiled expectantly, waiting for me to get it.

"Everything you see . . . is not that?" I asked, translating it literally. I thought for a moment. "Oh, like 'Nothing is as it appears,'" I said, laughing.

"Ah-*ha*!" he said, and laughed too. "Yes, Aaron!"

"Tout sa ou we . . ."

He nodded enthusiastically, grinning, waiting for me.

"One more time?" I asked him.

"*Se pa sa!*" he said. Then he repeated it once more. "*Tout sa ou we se pa sa!*"

"*Tout sa ou we se pa sa!*" I said slowly. "I think that's a good one for this situation, Père Eddy!"

He laughed again and then looked at me with earnest seriousness. "We will send a social worker from the mental health team to evaluate Janel so we can confirm he is able to consent for surgery and make sure he is prepared for this journey."

"That's a great idea," I said. "I think that would help him, and it would help us too. Thank you, Père Eddy."

"Thank *you*, Dr. Aaron, for standing in solidarity with this poor young man!" he said passionately. He smiled, grabbed my shoulder firmly, told me we'd keep in touch, and walked off.

I returned to the staff house from the hospital to pack my suitcase, lost in thought. I was hesitant. But Michelle, Anne, and now Père Eddy all thought there was no need to hesitate. We had funding. We had housing. And these two had led to hospital approval. Now all we needed was a visa. Martineau had said he was working on that. After months of overcoming various hurdles, we were finally close to achieving our goal of getting Janel the care he needed.

I should have been excited.

I should have been happy.

But I felt uneasy about the whole thing.

Waking up tangled in my mosquito net, soaked in sweat, my mouth parched, I saw it was still dark outside the small window over my bed. The electricity had gone off, waking me up as the fan spun its last few rotations, leaving the hot, humid air hanging heavy. The faint smoky smell of burning trash wafted in from outside. I wasn't sure if it was the silencing of the fan's hum that had woken me or the crowing roosters, barking dogs, and grunting pigs outside that had been masked by the whir of the fan before the power went out. *What time is it?* I wondered as I unraveled myself from my mosquito net. I was leaving that morning, and my ride to the airport was scheduled for 6 a.m. *Maybe it's almost that time anyway,* I thought.

I swung my legs over the side of the bed and peeled my sweat-soaked pajamas away from my skin. Standing and walking slowly with my hands held out in front of me, I felt for the room's small desk in the darkness. I made contact with the desk and patted across it with my hands, searching for my phone. I found it and pushed a button on it. Now a small square of light glowed in the darkness: 3:28 a.m. *Ugh.* The outdoor sounds seemed to be increasing in intensity. Or maybe I was just noticing them more. It seemed unlikely that I'd be able to fall back to sleep.

The light on my phone faded to black, plunging the room into darkness again. I noticed the odd feeling of something rubbery under my foot. Was it the edge of my flip-flop? No, it felt squishier than that. I pushed a button on my phone again for light and brought it down near the floor. A small yellow frog. I jumped back. It didn't seem to be moving. I nudged it gingerly with my toe. No response. I picked up my flip-flop from the floor and nudged the frog a bit more firmly with the edge of it. No response to that either. It was dead. Did it come into the room at night and die? Or did I step on it in the darkness and kill it? *I would've noticed that,* I thought.

I remembered seeing a frog perched in the corner of the shower the night before. I worried it would jump on me while I was showering, but it didn't. It never moved, and I wasn't sure if it was alive or dead. Was this the same one? I picked it up on the edge of my flip-flop and used my phone light to navigate my way out to the entrance of the house. It felt at least 10 degrees cooler outside. I tossed the frog into the darkness, came back into the stuffy heat of the house, and rinsed off my foot in the shower. I looked in the corner with my phone light. The frog was gone.

I lay back down on the bed and covered myself with my mosquito net. Half awake, I thought about Janel's bulging-eyed stare and Père Eddy's *Tout sa ou we se pa sa* and a dead yellow frog and about how I was sad to leave and glad to go home at the same time, dozing off for a few minutes here and there and then being awakened by a crowing rooster. *Can't they wait until dawn like they're supposed to?* I wondered. I turned over and tried to fall back to sleep.

By the time the driver picked me up at 6 a.m., the sun was coming up. As we drove through Mirebalais, there was already a lot of activity. Men in baseball caps herding cattle. Women carrying buckets, bins, and basins on their heads, bringing items to sell in the market or clothes to wash in the river.

As we navigated the winding mountain roads back to Port-au-Prince, the valleys below looked green and fertile beneath the morning mist, nothing like the barren, parched earth I had seen from the plane on the way in. After we arrived at the airport, I made my way through security to the departure gate.

Unlike my flight down to Haiti, on which I had seemed to be one of the only non-Haitian passengers, the gate for my return flight was filled with non-Haitians—mostly Americans. They stood out not only because they were nearly all white—almost nobody I'd seen for the last two weeks had been white—but also because they were often in large groups with matching T-shirts adorned with alliterative slogans on the front, like HELPING HAITI and HEALING HAITI and I ♥ HAITI and HAND IN HAND WITH HAITI and the clever IT'S A LOVE HAITI RELATIONSHIP. Many of the T-shirts had religious imagery or biblical quotations on the back. I wondered what these groups—many with school-age children—had been doing in Haiti.

I had overheard conversations in the Port-au-Prince airport and on flights to and from Haiti about people spending a week playing with children in an orphanage or laying a few bricks for a new church—what has come to be known as "voluntourism." For personal, religious, or other reasons, visiting volunteers have developed a desire to help those less fortunate than themselves. The intention is noble, but is a one-week volunteer trip truly helping Haitians or Haiti?

There are said to be more than 10,000 non-governmental organizations (NGOs) working in Haiti. That's one for every 1,000 people. And yet Haiti remains one of the poorest countries, with some of the worst health, education, and sanitation statistics in the world. Some organizations do phenomenal work helping individuals and communities. Yet their efforts are rarely coordinated with the government or one another, and funding comes and goes. Sometimes aid groups even do harm, unintentionally or, in the worst cases, intentionally.

Well-functioning organizations surely know how to incorporate short-term volunteers with no experience into projects in which their efforts can contribute toward some larger long-term goal. Yet I couldn't help but wonder if, instead of traveling to Haiti, it would be more helpful to have would-be voluntourists donate the price of their plane tickets to large humanitarian organizations with skills and experience in Haiti.

Adding up the 10 to 20 plane fares of a visiting spring-break crew . . . let's say conservatively at least $500 each, totaling $5,000 to $10,000 . . . and throwing in the cost of their matching T-shirts (or in one case, fleeces, though I've never experienced a temperature below 80 in Haiti—fleeces?) . . . let's say $40 each for another $400 to $800, the total amount could probably feed or provide medicine to a community for months, pay a schoolteacher's salary for a year, or provide loans for several local groups to start businesses. And that would be with the money from just one week of one program's flights and shirts.

But people want to go, to see, to experience. Bearing witness to poverty and suffering in Haiti and showing Haitians their solidarity could have positive effects beyond what can be measured or achieved through anonymous donations. And perhaps seeing firsthand how people live in Haiti inspires volunteers to open their hearts (and wallets) and encourage others to do the same in ways that reading about

Haiti in a book or news story cannot. But did these volunteer groups really see Haiti? Or did their hosting organizations show them a sugar-coated version, with performances by locals, intended to show how well their projects were functioning?

When I find myself being critical, I try to turn the same critique on myself to see if I am equally guilty of what I find myself criticizing in others. Seeing the extreme poverty of Haiti, and being only a neurologist, I sometimes feel I have little to offer. I hope my work will allow local doctors to take better care of their patients with neurologic diseases, but whether there is neurologic care in Haiti or not, Haiti will likely remain poor and politically unstable for the foreseeable future, with the majority of its citizens trapped in vicious cycles of poverty.

Of course I'm not trained to solve Haiti's economic, political, or social problems. I'm trained as a neurologist. If I can use my neurology training to the benefit of a few individuals while not causing any harm, and if I can work toward developing local capacity in neurology, perhaps I will accomplish some small good. Or should I be donating my plane fare to PIH instead of going to Haiti?

I was thinking about all of this as I boarded the plane and took my seat, which turned out to be next to Jack the plumber. In his late sixties, sporting a white handlebar mustache and a white ponytail, Jack had been coming to Haiti from Massachusetts for decades, supervising the plumbing construction and maintenance of nearly all the hospitals in the PIH/ZL network in Haiti. I often ran into him in the staff house at HUM, where we had enjoyed many dinner conversations.

"Fancy meeting you here, Aaron," he said with a smirk.

"Was about to make the same joke, Jack," I replied. "So what do you make of all these voluntourists with their matching Haiti T-shirts?" I smiled sarcastically. "What can a bunch of spring-break kids do down here anyway, right?"

I expected him to laugh and join in my critique. But he didn't. "You know what they can do, Aaron?" he said calmly but sternly. "They can haul buckets of concrete. They can dig a well or a latrine. I've seen it time and time again on project sites here. And many of them support the local economy, buying trinkets made by women in the villages and staying in Haitian hotels."

"Hmm," I said. Clearly I had been overly judgmental and critical without thinking through some of the potential positives. I took solace in the fact that I'd tried to be equally critical of myself.

"And you know what?" he continued. "A lot of them keep coming back. One of our best facilities engineers at HUM got hooked on Haiti after a high school mission trip way back, and now he works here most of the year."

"I didn't think about it that way," I conceded.

"Look, I know some of these organizations are just making a buck on a few tourists thinking they did something in Haiti when they really just goofed off and drank Prestige and Barbancourt," he said and chuckled, citing Haiti's local beer and rum brands. "But the big organizations are not beyond reproach. Did you ever read *Travesty in Haiti*?"

"I have it, but I haven't read it yet," I said. "I know the gist, though." The book is an exposé of corruption in the aid industry in Haiti—its subtitle is *A True Account of Christian Missions, Orphanages, Fraud, Food Aid, and Drug Trafficking*. "You're making me rethink this." I smiled at him.

"The doctors and nurses who come down here always say stuff like that," he said, smiling back. "I get it. But you know what I say? I say before we criticize the people who actually come down here to try to help, we should criticize the people who *don't*."

5

Applying for a visa requires a passport. Janel didn't have one. Applying for a passport requires some form of identification. Janel didn't have that either. Not even a birth certificate. As Martineau put it, Janel was so poor he had no proof that he existed.

Haiti is the poorest country in the Western Hemisphere, a distinction noted so frequently when Haiti is mentioned in the press that "the poorest country in the Western Hemisphere" has been referred to as Haiti's last name. But what does it actually mean to be the poorest country in a hemisphere? By the numbers, Haiti's GDP per capita—its national income divided by its number of citizens—is only $766 per person per year. That's about $2 per person per day. For comparison, the US GDP per capita is about $60,000 per person per year—about $164 per person per day—more than eighty times higher. But Haiti's GDP is not evenly distributed across its population. There are a few who are very rich and the vast majority is very poor. Being born in Haiti means an average life expectancy of sixty-four years, sixteen years shorter than the US average, even though the distance from Haiti to Miami is just half the distance from Miami to New York.

As tragic as these numbers are, they don't capture the human face of this poverty, faces like Janel's that become anonymous in these statistics. No passport means no visa. No birth certificate means no passport. And where do you stand in society if you can't even prove that you were born?

After Martineau first met Janel and saw his CT scan, he thought nothing could be done for him—certainly nothing in Haiti. When I told Martineau that not only was treatment possible but we had figured out how to get it for free in the US, he was determined to do whatever it took to get Janel a passport. But Martineau knew all too well how hard it was to navigate the bureaucracy required to obtain a passport in Haiti. He had recently missed the chance to go to a conference in the US because he wasn't able to get his own passport issued in time. It hadn't been for a lack of trying.

"In Haiti, everything you do, you need a *paren*," Martineau told me. "A *paren* literally means 'godfather' or 'godmother,' but it can also mean someone who is there to advocate for you—whether you need to buy a ticket at the airport, find a good school for your child, or even get the certificate that says you exist in this country. You can't do it without a *paren*. It's the Haitian reality."

It took months for Martineau to get a passport with his national identity card—not to mention his education, his position in society as a doctor, and his car to go back and forth to the immigration office. How would he even start the process for Janel if Janel had no form of identification?

Martineau discussed the situation with Michelle when she was in Haiti, but she wasn't sure how to help. One of the HUM administrators overheard their conversation. He mentioned that he had several contacts in various governmental posts who were part of the same masonic order as the one he belonged to, a spiritual group called L'Ancien et Mystique Ordre de la Rose-Croix (The Ancient and Mystical Order of the Rose-Cross). He assured Martineau that his contacts could help expedite Janel's passport. But this didn't solve the problem of finding some form of identification to start the process.

Martineau visited a local government office and tried to use his influence as a doctor caring for a local patient to plead his case for issuing an identity card for Janel without a birth certificate. The government official there offered to help if Martineau could provide proof of Janel's baptism. Unfortunately, if this proof once existed, it had been destroyed in a fire in Janel's childhood home. Wilner, the man who had taken Janel in, was a prominent member in his church. He was able to convince the church to provide a new baptism certificate for Janel. Martineau returned to the government office with this certificate, and they produced the documentation necessary to apply for a national identification card.

Documents in hand, Martineau drove to Port-au-Prince, where the well-connected HUM administrator had arranged appointments for him with contacts at the Office National d'Identification (ONI). The original ONI building had been destroyed in the 2010 earthquake, so the department was being run out of a house in a wealthy residential neighborhood of Port-au-Prince, an area of mansions, the Marriott, and the empty lot where the Sacré-Coeur cathedral had stood before it too was destroyed in the earthquake.

Martineau drove past multilevel houses surrounded by high concrete walls, bougainvillea flowers spilling over their tops between coils of barbed wire. He parked his car across the street from ONI in front of a tall metal gate, above which he could see the top floors of a large, luxurious house. An ambulance from HUM had brought Janel from Mirebalais to meet him there. Martineau and the ambulance driver slung Janel's arms over their shoulders and walked him into the temporary ONI facility.

Inside, they found themselves in a small concrete room with two people working at computers set up on a folding table. They sat Janel in a folding chair, and Martineau provided the information necessary to register Janel in their system. Janel sat silently, staring straight ahead, his hands now trembling nearly continuously.

The next step was to bring Janel to have a passport photo taken. But when Martineau exited ONI, a well-dressed light-skinned woman with blond highlights in her hair was standing in front of his car, hands on her hips.

"How dare you park in front of my gate!?" she yelled at him as he approached. "I have an ill family member inside who could die from being stuck in there!"

Martineau politely apologized, told her it was an emergency, and drove off.

"If it happens again, you'll end up with a flat tire!" she yelled after him.

As he drove to the photo booth, Martineau thought of going back and offering his services as a doctor to the sick person in the house. But he also couldn't help but wonder if the woman had made up the story for effect. A jolt interrupted his reflections as his car slammed to a halt.

He hopped out of the car to find his right front tire buried to the hubcap in an uncovered sewer drain. Two young boys who were waiting for shoe-shining customers on the curb across the street ambled over. Three teenagers followed behind them, their clothes tattered, their falling-apart flip-flops dangling from their feet. They were part of the legions of homeless young men who ran out into traffic and tried to wash windshields before the cars began moving again, then begged for money for their services. The five boys told Martineau to get back into his car and put it in reverse while they pushed and lifted the front of his car out of the sewer drain. Somehow it worked, and Martineau gave them each a few dollars. The tire was ruined, but the photo booth was less than a block away.

Martineau was determined to get Janel's picture before dealing with the tire. He and the ambulance driver brought Janel into the photo booth and dressed him in a suit jacket they had found in the photo booth's costume closet. Once Janel's picture was taken, the ambulance took him back to Mirebalais.

Martineau flagged down a motorcyclist and paid him for a ride to the nearest car repair shop. While the motorcycle driver waited there, Martineau purchased a tire from the auto mechanic. He then flagged down a second motorcycle. The repair shop's mechanic mounted the second motorcycle, sandwiched the tire between himself and the driver, and they followed Martineau's motorcycle ride back to his car.

While Martineau and the mechanic toiled to replace the tire in the midday heat, cars and motorcycles zipping past them, Martineau received a call from his well-connected colleague in the HUM administration. His colleague's contact at the Ministry of the Interior—who happened to be the minister himself—could meet Martineau that afternoon, but only if Martineau could arrive in the next hour.

Martineau had never met a government official before. He looked down at his grease-streaked hands, sweat-soaked button-down shirt, and casual loafers. "I'm not dressed to meet a minister," Martineau said to him. "I don't even have socks on today!"

His colleague laughed. "No problem. He's waiting for you." He hung up.

Once the tire was replaced, Martineau paid the mechanic and the two motorcycle drivers. He then drove to the Ministry of the Interior, about fifteen minutes away. When he arrived, security guards led him to an extravagant hotel-like lobby, where light-skinned secretaries dressed in chic, tightly fitting dresses and high heels greeted him and escorted him to the office of the minister.

The minister sat behind an elegant wooden desk equipped with several computers that looked to Martineau to be the latest models. He had one cell phone in each hand. He was wearing a tan-and-white checkered sport coat over a light blue shirt, the top few buttons of which were open, revealing a thick gold chain. His hair was closely cropped, and he was clean-shaven except for a perfectly groomed slim mustache that traced the angle of his upper lip. Smiling down from the wall behind the minister's desk was an enormous photographic portrait of President Michel Martelly. The portrait was dominated by Martelly's glistening shaven head, which had given rise to his party's name, Tèt Kale (Bald Headed). The president's dark blue suit and the red-and-blue presidential sash across his chest disguised his origins as the *kompa* singer Sweet Micky, (in)famous for performing in a miniskirt, a diaper, or nothing at all, for mooning, punching, and propositioning his audience members, and for smoking crack cocaine.

The minister waved Martineau in and motioned for him to sit down.

Martineau introduced himself as a doctor in Mirebalais and a colleague of the HUM administrator who'd set up the appointment.

"Kouman m ka aide ou jodi a la, Dok?" asked the minister. ("How can I help you today, Doc?")

Martineau explained that he had a young patient with a large brain tumor who needed surgery in the US, and a team in Boston had agreed to do the surgery for free. The patient needed a passport as soon as possible so he could get a visa to go to the US for the operation. Would the minister be so kind as to help expedite the passport process?

With a brisk nod, the minister used one of his cell phones to begin calling colleagues in the immigration office. While the minister was on the phone, Martineau looked around the office, impressed with its luxuriousness. *So this is how things happen in Haiti when you are rich and connected,* he mused. Maybe with such connections, he thought, he would have been able to get his passport in time to make it to the conference he had wanted to attend in the US a few months ago. And maybe he wouldn't have nearly died when he was fourteen years old.

Martineau was born with some swelling in his groin, diagnosed as a congenital inguinal hernia. His mother heard about a group of visiting American surgeons and was able to get him a hernia repair operation for free when he was still a baby. But the surgery failed, and three days later, the hernia recurred. Since he had no symptoms from it aside from mild swelling in his groin, he and his family ignored it.

Martineau's mother moved with him and his sister to Port-au-Prince, hoping to find a job there. She didn't find one. Instead, she sold water. Each day she walked to a small spring about two miles outside the city, filled a bucket, carried it back on her head, and went from door to door in their neighborhood, selling the water. When the bucket was empty, she went back to the spring, brought a newly filled bucket back on her head, and continued making her way through the neighborhood.

She went back and forth to the spring more than ten times every day. The other children in the neighborhood teased Martineau for being the son of the water seller—even among the poor, he was considered poor. Martineau, his sister, and his mother shared one room in a small three-room concrete house with a tin roof, and his family ate two meals a day: breakfast was a cup of strong coffee to try to stave off hunger until the afternoon meal.

When Martineau was seven years old, his mother withdrew him from school so she could try to get him another surgery for the hernia. Every day for several weeks, Martineau and his mother made the thirty-minute trip to the General Hospital of Port-au-Prince in the back of an overcrowded *taptap* and waited among large crowds outside, hoping to get an appointment. Unable to read or write, Martineau's mother had difficulty navigating the hospital. At one point she managed to meet a young woman surgeon who promised she would try to help them. They met with her twice, but then they never saw her again. Martineau's mother thought it was because the doctor knew she couldn't afford the surgery. Dispirited, she gave up.

At age fourteen, Martineau awoke one Sunday morning and vomited. He had his morning coffee and vomited again. He noticed his groin was even more swollen than usual. Then his abdomen began to distend like a balloon about to burst. Over the course of the morning, he began vomiting uncontrollably. His mother took him back to the General Hospital by *taptap*. This time it was an emergency, and they didn't need to wait in line. He was rushed to surgery. Martineau's intestines had become entrapped in the hernia—incarcerated, in medical terminology—and sections of his bowel had begun to die, a condition that can be fatal if not treated promptly.

Telling Janel's story to the minister had reminded Martineau that at one point he had not been so different from Janel: a poor boy in need of surgery but with no money or connections to make it happen. Perhaps if there had been someone to advocate for him, he wouldn't have lived for fourteen years with the ticking time bomb of an unrepaired hernia and wouldn't have nearly died when his bowels became strangulated in it. And here he was, providing that very advocacy for Janel, giving, in his words, "a voice to the voiceless" and being "a defender of the weak."

"I was thinking that although I did not have the opportunity to get the care I needed until it was nearly too late," he later told me, "somehow the universe offered me the possibility to offer this opportunity to someone else."

The minister hung up the phone, smiled, and said the immigration office would be expecting Martineau the next day. On the back of his business card, he wrote the phone number of a colleague who worked there and handed the card to Martineau. Martineau accepted it gingerly with both hands as if he'd been given a precious jewel, and he thanked the minister for his kindness. As Martineau left the lavish office, he was amazed at how seemingly easy it was to navigate the Haitian system when you knew people in power.

Martineau awoke the next morning to news that anti-government protests were scheduled in Port-au-Prince not far from the immigration office. A government stalemate had delayed parliamentary elections, raising concerns that President Martelly could rule by decree. Protesters were demanding that he and his prime minister resign. Driving through mass protests in Port-au-Prince means risking having one's car windows broken by rock-throwing protesters or, worse, having the car set on fire.

Martineau parked at the immigration office and walked through the masses of people assembled on its grounds. He described the scene to me as "exactly in the image of Haiti": poor people who can't read or write spending months there without getting an appointment, rich people walking in and out with their papers on the same day, and hustlers looking to cheat the vulnerable poor.

After several failed attempts at reaching the minister's contact by phone, Martineau finally succeeded and was told to meet the official in his office up a set of stairs. But security guards at the top of the staircase refused to let him enter, and despite several attempts to call his contact, Martineau again couldn't reach him.

Martineau remembered he had the business card of the minister of the interior in his wallet, and showed it to the guards. As if he'd said the magic word, they opened the doors and escorted him into a smoke-filled suite, where the faces of political figures he recognized from television and newspapers appeared to float in the haze emanating from their cigarettes.

Martineau provided the minister's contact with the paperwork from ONI and the photo of Janel from the day before. Thirty minutes later, he left with Janel's passport in his hands. What had taken him months to do for himself through the normal mechanisms—normal at least for those who can read and write—had taken about forty-eight hours with connections to the right people.

Janel now had proof that he existed.

The visa process was much simpler. Back in Boston, Anne filled out an online form for a medical emergency visa for Janel on the website of the US embassy in Haiti, and the appointment was granted a few days later. Anne and I wrote a letter of medical necessity committing to provide all care free of charge and got it signed by Brigham and PIH. Martineau took this letter, the visa fee, and Janel to the consulate and received the visa within hours.

Anne and I asked the Brigham admitting office to book a bed on the neurology ward, the neurosurgery team to book an operating room slot in the following week, and the Ray Tye Medical Aid Foundation to book a medical flight for Janel on an air ambulance.

On December 24, Martineau arrived at the Port-au-Prince airport at sunrise with Janel and his mother in an HUM ambulance. An airport official escorted the vehicle directly onto the tarmac, where the medical flight awaited. A young, blond flight nurse stepped off the plane in a one-piece zip-up uniform that Martineau thought looked like a space suit. She greeted Martineau, asked him about Janel's medical condition, did a brief physical examination, and then loaded Janel onto a stretcher.

"I felt like a hero at that moment," Martineau later told me, "because I followed the patient through the whole process. It felt like an extraordinary accomplishment. I felt proud of myself, but I also thought: I did not deny my origins. What happens most of the time to the middle class in Haiti is that once they come from the rural regions to Port-au-Prince and they succeed, then they completely forget their origins, their roots. So in my case, thanks to God, I didn't have that problem. I know my origin. And so I think it's normal that I help poor people who are like how I was."

Martineau looked at Janel's mother as she watched the air ambulance crew load Janel's stretcher onto the plane. He wondered what this all looked like to her. She had arrived at the airport in Haiti's largest city from a wooden hut in a region so rural that there were no roads, and was now seeing an airplane for what was probably the first time, an airplane that would take her child to *lòt bò a*—the other side.

"Was she sad to see him leave?" I later asked Martineau. "Was she afraid?"

"She wasn't sad. I think she was moved, but she didn't cry. She was really strong. She was very proud, because Janel had found a solution. Because the Haitian mentality is that if you receive something from foreigners, it is something good. So, far from having fear, I saw hope in her face."

6

While Janel was in the air, I was seeing neurology consults at Brigham with a team of residents and students. My phone chirped throughout the day with one-line updates from the air ambulance team by email:

> 10:35 a.m. We have landed in Haiti and will update you once we have made patient contact.

> 11:19 a.m. We have the patient loaded onto the aircraft and we are departing Haiti.

> 2:09 p.m. We have landed at our fuel stop in Jacksonville, FL, and everything is going well.

> 2:56 p.m. We have cleared customs, fueled, and are now departing Jacksonville, FL.

And when I asked how Janel was doing, they wrote:

> My medical team said the patient is awake and enjoying all of our snacks that we have on the plane.

I forwarded these to Michelle as they came in.
"Woohoo!! Love the play by play!!" she wrote back.

"I know, I guess that's what $33,000 gets you!" I replied, citing the cost of the medical flight that the Ray Tye Medical Aid Foundation had generously paid for.

"Madness . . . This is also why poverty is so debilitating," she responded.

We received our final update around 5:30 p.m.:

> We have arrived at Bedford, MA, and will be going bedside
> with the patient shortly.

I updated Michelle and Hermide, and we planned to meet at Brigham later in the evening. Anne was working and couldn't join us. It had been a busy day and I wanted to spend time with Janel when he arrived, so I walked home to have a quick dinner with Nina. At that time, we lived about a twenty-five-minute walk from Brigham. Bedford is about twenty miles from Boston, so I figured that between rush-hour traffic and the time it would take the nurses to get Janel settled in his hospital bed, the timing should work out perfectly.

Just as we sat down to eat, I heard the piercing electronic beeping of my pager. It wasn't uncommon for me to get paged at home when I was on the consult service. Doctors from other teams who consulted us had questions, and residents called to discuss patients they had seen. But this page wasn't about the consult service. It was from the neurology resident who would be taking care of Janel when he arrived. I had spoken with him about the plan for Janel before leaving the hospital. Presuming he just had some questions for me since Janel had no medical records in our system, I went into the bedroom to call him back.

"What's up?" I asked.

"The nurses on the floor said your guy from Haiti blew a pupil and they're sending him to the emergency room," he said.

My stomach dropped like I was on a roller coaster in free fall. A blown pupil is a dilated pupil that won't react to light. It's an ominous sign suggesting intracranial pressure—the pressure inside the skull—is high enough that the brain is pressing on one of the nerves that controls the size of the pupil.

"What?!" I shouted into the phone.

"I don't know, they just said—"

"On my way," I interrupted, and hung up before he could answer.

I ran past the kitchen to grab my coat and workbag.

"Everything okay?" Nina asked.

"Sorry, gotta go back to the hospital," I called from across the apartment. "Sounds like Janel's in bad shape."

"Oh no! You want a ride? I can pick you up when you're finished."

"No, I'll just jog over. I suspect it's going to be a late night."

"It's raining out. You should drive."

I looked outside. It had begun pouring. I shook my head.

Nina brought me the car keys. "I hope he's okay," she said, her eyes moving back and forth across my panicked expression.

"Yeah . . . I'll let you know," I said, distracted, frazzled, wondering what I had gotten myself into.

"Drive safe," she called after me as I ran out through the rain to the car.

My heart was racing as I began driving back to Brigham. One of many worst-case scenarios I had worried about in thinking through Janel's care was the possibility of something bad happening on the plane. Because his tumor blocked the passages between the fluid-filled ventricles of his brain, the ventricles had expanded due to the backup of flow, a condition called hydrocephalus—literally "water head." Although our abdomens easily expand after each meal to accommodate the food we have eaten, the rigid skull is a much less forgiving space. Even slight increases in pressure in or around the brain can lead to intense headaches, nausea, and vomiting. Severely elevated intracranial pressure can cause coma or even death.

Just as water bottles hiss when opened on a plane and shampoo bottles pop open in checked baggage, flying at altitude in a pressurized cabin could cause Janel's already-elevated intracranial pressure to rise further. I had found that the World Health Organization website listed increased intracranial pressure as a contraindication to air travel. When I mentioned my concern to Ian—the neurosurgeon who would be operating on Janel—and one of my senior neurology colleagues at Brigham, they thought the risk was more of a theoretical one, unlikely to actually affect the patient. But we hadn't wanted to take any chances. We had asked the Ray Tye Medical Aid Foundation not only to hire an air ambulance for Janel but to pay the extra fee for one that could fly near sea level without pressurizing the cabin.

As I pulled up to a red light, I wondered if I could run it and flash my medical badge to a police officer if I got pulled over, something I'd never tried or needed to do before. But I figured it would only take me even longer to get to Brigham if I got pulled over, even if they let me go without a ticket when I explained the situation. I stopped at the light, but my mind sped ahead.

The messages from the flight crew had said that Janel was fine. But a blown pupil suggested something catastrophic. What had happened? The windshield wipers whipping back and forth in the heavy rain made me think of the rhythm of chest compressions performed when attempting to resuscitate a dying patient.

I imagined Janel unconscious on a stretcher in the middle of a code blue. One doctor compressing Janel's sternum vigorously with one palm over the other, her white coat flapping behind her. Another doctor tilting Janel's head back, prying his jaw open, and snaking a breathing tube down his throat. Nurses putting IVs into his arms and shouting out vital signs. Monitors beeping. Pagers going off. A doctor standing at the foot of the bed calmly but firmly summarizing what had been done so far and what was to be done next, trying to be heard over the commotion. And the on-call neurosurgeon hovering impatiently in the corner, arms crossed, waiting to get Janel to the operating room.

What if Janel had developed some complication en route that made his tumor inoperable? What if he died soon after arriving at Brigham? After all we had done to get him to Boston . . .

The light changed to green. I sped toward Brigham, crookedly parallel parked on a side street near the hospital, threw my workbag over my shoulder, jumped out of the car, slammed the door, and ran through the pouring rain toward the six illuminated Greek columns of the 15 Francis Street entrance to the hospital.

This entrance put me at one end of a long hallway that leads to the main entrance at 75 Francis Street, where the emergency room is. I jogged down the hallway, raindrops flying off my jacket, my workbag slapping against my back.

I arrived in the emergency room out of breath and noticed a group of several nurses, doctors, and staff outside a curtained-off area in the far corner. A crowd in a hospital is generally a bad sign. I began frantically weaving between gurneys and computer workstations to get across the emergency room. I made my way to the back of the curtained-off area and peeked inside, expecting to see a blur of white coats swarming around the small space.

Instead, I saw only Janel on a gurney.

He was rolled onto his right side and in the fetal position, looking at the wall with his wide-eyed stare. He was wearing the same tan suit as when I had met him a few weeks earlier in Haiti. Despite the big crowd outside the curtain, nobody was inside the curtained-off area except him. *If he's alone in here*, I thought, *he must be okay.*

I stepped in and closed the curtain. I squatted down between the wall he was facing and the gurney so we were eye to eye. The commotion of the emergency room—charged conversations, chirping monitors, beeping pagers, overhead announcements, ambulance sirens—faded into the background.

Inside the curtain, it felt quiet.

Janel and I stared at each other.

My heart was still racing, both from fear and from running through the hospital to the emergency room. But Janel seemed to be all right. My level of panic began to subside.

"*W sonje'm?*" I asked him. ("Do you remember me?")

He stared at me and blinked once, slowly. *"Wi"* ("Yes"), he responded softly in his high-pitched raspy voice, without a hint of facial expression. He looked the same as he had a few weeks before in Haiti. I took a penlight out of my workbag and shined it in each eye. His pupils were indeed different sizes, the right one slightly larger than the left. Neither constricted in response to the light as it should. Had I even examined his pupils in Haiti? Or had I been too shocked that he didn't look like the twenty-three-year-old college student I had imagined and neglected to examine him as closely as I should have? I couldn't remember. The tumor was pressing on the region of his brain that controls the pupils, so it was certainly reasonable to expect they wouldn't work properly. They probably hadn't for a long time.

I took a deep breath and let it out slowly. He looked fine. He looked fine! Well, not fine, of course, but he was not in some sort of acute neurologic crisis as I'd feared. I started to settle into relief, and time began to slow back to its normal pace after the frenetic last fifteen minutes since my pager had gone off.

"W te renmen avion an?" I asked, smiling. ("Did you like the airplane?") I wasn't sure what else to say.

He stared at me. *"Wi,"* he eked out after a pause, expressionless.

As I began to relax, it dawned on me: He was here. *Lòt bò a*—the other side. *He made it!* I smiled. Several months, hundreds of emails later, Janel was in Boston. *We did it!*

I stayed there squatting in front of Janel for a moment, overwhelmed by the sudden convergence of the two disparate worlds I had been traveling between: the high-tech wealth and comfort of Boston and the devastating poverty and suffering of rural Haiti. Seeing Janel in front of me at Brigham, I was deeply moved by what PIH was able to achieve for their patients, and grateful for the chance to play some small role in their mission.

"Tann mwen yon ti moman," I said, patting him gently on the hand. ("I'll be back in a minute.")

I stepped outside the curtain and recognized an emergency room doctor I knew. He was talking to a young woman who must have been one of the flight nurses, judging by her space-suit-like red-and-blue uniform. A few other nurses and staff stood around them.

They looked at me, surprised, not expecting someone to emerge from behind the curtain.

"I'm one of the doctors who helped bring him here from Haiti," I said. "He looks the same as he did a few weeks ago when I was there. How did he end up in the emergency room?"

The flight nurse laughed. "His pupils are two different sizes," she said. "When I told the nurse on the ward, she panicked and told us to send him to the emergency room. I told her that his pupils were like that even before we took off and that I wasn't concerned, but she insisted."

I nodded.

"Honestly," she said, lowering her voice, "I think it was just the end of her shift and she didn't want to deal with this complicated new patient." She laughed again.

I turned to the emergency room doctor. "Sounds like a false alarm," I said. "We already have a bed ready on the neurology floor. Can we send him up directly?"

"Sounds like a plan to me," he responded. "We'll call transport." He walked away to one of the computer workstations, and the other staff dispersed.

"Oh," I called after him, "can you not log this as an emergency visit so it's not billed?"

He looked over his shoulder quizzically and then shrugged. "Sure," he called back. An emergency room visit can lead to a bill of thousands of dollars. That wasn't part of our budget estimate for Janel's care.

I turned back to the flight nurse in her red-and-blue space suit.

"Thanks for bringing him," I said and smiled.

"It's so amazing you could get him here for surgery," she said, smiling back.

"Well, it's been a huge team effort . . ." I began.

"Yes!" she said excitedly, grabbing my arm. "Oh my gosh, Dr. Martineau—what an amazing guy! He came right with the patient onto the tarmac and spoke such perfect English. We donated a whole bunch of extra medical supplies we had on board to him to take back to the hospital where he works."

"Martineau is amazing," I said. "And we couldn't have done it without you!" I thanked her and we exchanged email addresses so I could let her know how Janel did.

The transport team came to bring Janel to the neurology ward. I walked with them as they wheeled his gurney to the elevators. As we ascended, I wondered if Janel had ever been in an elevator before. Probably not. His fixed wide-eyed stare made him look perpetually afraid, so it was hard to tell what his reaction was to all of the activity around him in this new and strange place. His first view of the US was the high-tech and frenetic environment of a hospital emergency room. Not exactly the Statue of Liberty, the Grand Canyon, or Disney World.

We arrived on the tenth floor and steered Janel's gurney to his room. The room was only slightly larger than the hospital bed at its center, a chair next to it, and a small sink in the corner. A TV screen was mounted on the wall. Outside the window, tiny blurred red and white points glimmered in the rainy darkness, the lights of cars on the streets down below. The nurses aligned the gurney parallel to the hospital bed, brought down its side railing, and pulled the sheet with Janel on it onto the bed. He lay there, motionless, blinking occasionally. I sat down in the chair next to him.

What was he thinking? What did it all look like to him? Was it as exotic and fascinating and confusing and mysterious as his country had seemed to me when I first visited? Was he afraid? Was he just a quiet guy? I wanted to ask him these questions. I wanted to make sure he understood what was going to be happening and to reassure him that we'd take good care of him. I suppose I just wanted to connect with him in some way. I was, after all, only thirteen years older than he was.

We sat in silence until I thought of a simple question I knew how to ask in Creole. *"W grangou?"* ("Are you hungry?")

He raised his eyebrows very slightly while slowly making a small nod upward of his chin. It was the first facial expression of any kind that I'd seen him make. I presumed it meant yes.

Finally, here was something I could do for him. I took the hospital menu and translated each item into Creole.

"Do you want chicken?"

He closed his eyes and lifted his right hand an inch off the bed, slightly straightening his fingers. His hand began trembling and he put it back down. Seemed like a no.

"Beef?"

He closed his eyes.

"Spaghetti?"

He closed his eyes again.

"Fish?"

Same gesture.

"Salad? . . . Chips? . . . Fruit? . . . Cake? . . . Cookies?"

No to all of these. I went back to the top.

"Chicken?"

He raised his eyebrows slightly. Yes? Maybe?

I smiled. "Chicken, then?"

He closed his eyes.

This was going to be harder than I thought. Was it my Creole? Was there just nothing on the menu he wanted? Was he completely overwhelmed? Was the tumor putting so much pressure on his brain that he couldn't process what was happening?

I ordered him a few different things and turned on the television. Channel by channel I asked if he liked the show or movie. He stared intently at the television but made the closed-eyed no gesture to every channel when I asked him if he wanted to keep watching it.

We continued this confusing exchange for a few minutes until I heard *"Kouman ou ye!?!"* ("How are you!?!") half shouted, half sung from the doorway. I turned around to see Michelle in an orange-and-black plaid peacoat, smiling broadly. We hugged tightly, shaking our heads, amazed that Janel was actually here. She set a chocolate croissant and a bottle of soda in front of him. I thought I saw the faintest suggestion of a smile at the corners of his mouth, but I wasn't sure if I was imagining it.

Michelle asked Janel if he'd like to try the croissant. He didn't respond. She broke off a piece and gently fed it to him. Janel chewed it for a few moments and then closed his eyes and made the subtlest hint of a grimace.

Michelle laughed. *"W pa renmen'l?"* ("You don't like it?")

He closed his eyes, frowned slightly, and raised one tremulous hand a few inches off the bed.

"I've been striking out on trying to figure out food too," I told her.

She laughed again.

The door opened and Hermide entered. "Helloooooooo!" she exclaimed gleefully with a flourish of her hands as she came through the door with several friends. Hermide was in her late sixties, but her luminous eyes and radiant smile made her look much younger, as did her stylish wig—a light brown, face-framing, chin-length bob with angled bangs. The deep creases around her mouth and under her eyes were the only clues to her age.

"This must be Janel," she said with the slight lilt of a Caribbean accent, pronouncing his name softly and deeply, with reverence. She moved toward him with a serene smile and wide-open arms. He didn't react. She converted what was intended to be a hug to simply putting her hands gently on his cheeks. It looked like the scene of a mother reuniting with her reluctant long-estranged son: love and anticipation on one side, aloof ambivalence on the other. This didn't seem to bother Hermide. She excitedly began unpacking containers of Haitian food she had made for him, naming each dish as she put it out: *diri ak sos pwa* (rice with bean sauce), *poule* (chicken), *legim* (vegetable stew). She opened one container and began feeding him, dabbing his mouth gently and lovingly with a napkin between bites.

The room was filled with the sounds of Haitian Creole as Michelle talked to Hermide and her friends. I struggled to pick up bits and pieces, laughing when they laughed even if I didn't understand. Janel stared straight ahead while Hermide fed him, not speaking or interacting with anyone. Eventually we decided we should let him rest, and we departed. We waved goodbye. He didn't react, continuing to stare at the television, where *Spider-Man* was playing.

Michelle and I rode the elevator down to the hospital lobby. "You did it!" she said and smiled.

"Come on, *we* did it!" I said.

We high-fived, beaming.

"This has been like a second full-time job," I said, shaking my head. "I had no idea . . ."

"Welcome to my world!" she said and laughed.

The elevator doors opened, and we stepped into the high-ceilinged lobby, empty at this late hour. We looked at each other, smiled, and shook our heads.

"It's so crazy to see him here in Boston and think about where he came from," she said. "That area in Haiti where he lives is so poor." She looked away for a moment, and I thought I recognized the look in her eyes that I imagined I had when I thought about Haiti from afar.

I was starting to have that movie-happy-ending emotion somewhere between wanting to cry and wanting to laugh. "It feels like we just had a baby or something," I said and chuckled.

"About as much struggle and about as much joy to see him on the other side, right!?" she quipped back.

We hugged, said good night, and went our separate ways. I drove back up the same street I had driven down in a panic a few hours earlier. Now I felt elated. Janel had gone from rural Haiti—without even a birth certificate to prove he existed—to a Harvard hospital for care by a renowned neurosurgeon by way of an air ambulance. I couldn't believe we had pulled this off.

When I arrived home, I found I had received an email from the flight nurse with pictures attached, some aerial views of Haiti and a picture of Martineau giving a thumbs-up from the tarmac as the plane took off.

> Please extend my deepest gratitude to the donors that made this possible! I was so moved! Thank you for the opportunity to serve this family and your team. Please let me know his condition if you have time. My family and I are praying for him.
>
> P.S. I spoke with my mother via text telling her why I would not be home for Christmas and it was the best Christmas ever! This is what she sent. . . .
>
>> "The two most important days of your life are the day you are born, and the day you find out why."—Mark Twain. You are one of those rare people who discovered what your "why" is . . . a blessing to many. Stay safe.
>
> She is right: we are so blessed!

It was inspiring to see her and her mother so touched by Janel and his story. After months of negotiating, worrying, strategizing, and questioning, somehow it all felt right—so right others could see it too. No talk of cost-effectiveness or sustainability here. The flight nurse and her mother saw what I saw: A young man with a debilitating neurologic disease who had every right to healthcare but no access to it. The poverty and suffering in Haiti just a short flight away from our shores. And how working together, maybe we could do something about it, one patient at a time.

7

Janel yawned deeply, his head rolling slowly back in his wheelchair until he nearly bumped into the kitsch painting of sailboats hanging on the wall behind him.

"I guess that can serve as our airway exam," the anesthesiologist said as she chuckled, referring to the need for a preoperative examination of the back of the throat. She would be the doctor passing the breathing tube into Janel's lungs after putting him under in the operating room.

We were assembled in what we call the "family meeting room," a small wood-paneled conference room just down the hall from the hospital ward where patients and their families can convene with the medical staff in a quieter and more comfortable setting than the small patient rooms. Countless times as a resident, I had sat with expectant families in this room and others like it to provide updates on their loved ones' condition, to present bad news, or to discuss difficult choices.

Today, none of the individuals in the room with Janel were members of his family. The group consisted of the anesthesia team, Janel's nurse, a Haitian Creole interpreter, a social worker, Hermide, and me. Neurosurgeon Ian Dunn was on his way. The room was just barely large enough to accommodate the oblong Formica conference table and everyone sitting around it.

As we waited for Ian, I wondered what it all looked like to Janel. It had been about a week since his first plane ride, his first elevator ride. We still hadn't exchanged more than a few words despite my daily visits to his hospital room. Michelle, Anne, and Hermide hadn't had better luck even with their fluent Creole.

I prided myself on being able to make some kind of connection with most of my patients, especially my Haitian American patients in Boston, whose expressions often brightened when they heard I could produce a few phrases in Creole. I hadn't expected to become friends with Janel. He would see me as his doctor and would presumably want me to see him as my patient. But I found it challenging to know how to approach the little details of his comfort and the larger aspects of his care without being able to communicate with him. I wasn't sure what he understood, what he wanted, what he needed, what he expected, what he hoped for.

Why didn't he talk to us? Was it his brain tumor? His personality? The disorientation of being alone in Boston, surrounded by strangers speaking English, looking out from a tenth floor window when he'd never left the ground before? We didn't know.

A social worker and psychiatrist from the mental health team at HUM had evaluated Janel before he came to Boston to make sure he truly understood the risks and benefits of surgery. They had told us he did and that a full report would follow. We had received the report a few days after Janel arrived at Brigham.

The social worker and psychiatrist had written that Janel didn't speak much, and when he did, he spoke slowly. They described Janel as "cooperative and endearing," frequently making eye contact with them. They described his cognition as "slowed and dulled" but reported that, in spite of this, his insight and judgment were "intact":

> *This young man reports that he is aware he has an illness in his head and that he requires a procedure for treatment. He recognizes that this illness is potentially fatal and that the intervention, while it has a likelihood of improving his health, carries significant risks, including death. Due to physical discomfort (he had significant pain in his head and needed to lie down often), we were not able to speak*

with him at length. However, he explained that his religious faith
keeps him going, and that he remains hopeful about his future. He
continues to pray daily.

  In terms of capacity, he was able to confirm his understanding
of the surgical intervention, the risks and benefits, and his desire
to undergo the procedure. He also stated that he trusts Wilner
to speak on his behalf. We did not detect any evidence of mental
illness that interferes with his ability to make decisions on his
own. While his cognition is impaired due to physical illness, he is
coherent. Furthermore, he is reflective and self-aware and wishes to
participate in his medical care.

Michelle, Anne, Hermide, and I had difficulty imagining Janel communicating all of this, considering we had not heard any more than a
rare *"Wi"* ("Yes") from him since he had arrived. Maybe he was simply
more comfortable speaking openly in Haiti. We hoped this would
change as he got used to us, since he could be spending up to two
months in Boston.

The report concluded:

Despite the challenges his family faces related to living in rural
Haiti, he is embedded within a loving and supportive family
and community. Furthermore, he has been reflective about this
entire experience, suggesting psychological fortitude, and he is
expressing hopefulness for his future. Nonetheless, he is now
facing a life-changing event and intervention without any of these
supports physically present with him. Psychologically, this would
be potentially traumatizing for anyone. Therefore, every effort
should be made to strengthen and bolster his psychological and
social reserves.

Since we were having difficulty engaging with Janel, Michelle had
asked some young Haitian Americans who lived in Boston and worked

for her organization, EqualHealth, to come keep him company. One day a young woman about Janel's age was going through the TV channels with him, trying to find something he liked, as I'd done unsuccessfully on a few occasions.

She flipped to a cartoon channel. *"Dessin anime?"* she asked him.

A quick, small, once back-and-forth of his head. No.

The next channel had a high-speed car chase. *"Film d'action?"*

The same gesture. Another no.

She changed the channel again. An alien movie. *"Film extraterrestre?"* He closed his eyes. No again.

She flipped to the next channel. A soccer match. *"Football? Ou renmen football?"* She looked at him hopefully. Soccer is very popular in Haiti. Men crowd around small television sets in one-room restaurants to get a glimpse of a game, cheering wildly for their favorite teams.

Janel closed his eyes again.

She went to the next channel. A woman and man kissing with a swell of romantic music. *"Film d'amour?"* She looked at him and frowned, expecting a definite no to this one.

He smiled slightly and slowly began nodding his head up and down.

"Oooo ooo," she half sang, half squealed. *"Janel renmen film d'amour!"* she sang as if teasing a childhood friend on the playground. ("Janel likes romantic movies!")

Now he smiled fully at her. A broad smile, showing all of his bright white teeth, his lower lip jutting out and curling slightly as his smile grew. It was the first time I'd seen him make any substantial facial expression.

"W renmen film d'amour, Janel?" I asked, smiling and trying to join in the dialogue by repeating what the young woman had said. ("You like romantic movies, Janel?")

He turned his head slowly toward me, his smile taking on a more mischievous air. He quickly raised and lowered his eyebrows as he lifted his chin briskly upward.

There's a twenty-three-year-old boy in there after all! I thought. His smile slowly receded as he watched the movie, and he settled back into his usual, staring silence. It was the only moment that felt close to a meaningful interaction with him in the entire week he'd been in Boston.

The door to the family meeting room opened, and Ian Dunn appeared in blue scrubs and a long white coat. Although we had emailed each other, I'd never seen him before. He looked only a few years older than me, and yet he had a certain gravitas: tall, with a broad-shouldered athletic build, short dark blond hair graying at the temples combed to one side over a high forehead, and intensely focused dark blue eyes with light purple shadows beneath them. He walked with a clear sense of purpose as he made his way to the only open seat at the head of the table. I introduced myself and shook hands with him. My hand felt small compared to his and collapsed in his strong grip—a surgeon's handshake.

The social worker called Wilner in Haiti, put him on speakerphone, and asked everyone to introduce themselves. Then it was Ian's turn. He thanked all the members of the team. Speaking deliberately in a deep baritone, he explained that surgery was scheduled for two days later. He listed the risks of the operation as nonchalantly as if giving driving directions. "Bleeding, stroke, seizure, disability." He paused briefly. "Even death." Ian's face barely moved as he spoke except for a flicker of slight creases in his forehead from time to time. He paused after each line so the Creole interpreter could translate.

"However," he concluded matter-of-factly, "we believe the benefits of performing the surgery outweigh the risks, and we will do everything we can to minimize those risks."

Janel didn't look at Ian or anyone else. He sat expressionless, staring straight ahead, blinking occasionally.

Through a staticky connection, Wilner thanked everyone for their care of Janel. He affirmed his understanding and confirmed that he spoke on behalf of Janel and his family. He conveyed that his and their wishes were to do everything possible to treat Janel, acknowledging the risks. *"Kounyea se nan men Bondye,"* he said solemnly. The interpreter translated: "Now it's in the hands of God."

Ian rose from his position at the head of the table and stood to the right of Janel's wheelchair, towering over him. Janel continued to stare straight ahead. "I'm going to make an incision right here," Ian said, bending slightly forward and slowly tracing a line with his index finger from the base of Janel's skull several inches down his neck. I imagined his scalpel piercing the skin as an assistant dabbed at the line of blood following the tip of the blade. If Janel understood the gesture, he didn't react.

"Any questions?" Ian asked. He pulled up a chair next to Janel and sat down. He took a sheet of paper from his white coat pocket and placed it on the table in front of Janel: the consent form, a standard document with spaces to fill in for the doctor's name, the operation to be performed, the risks of the procedure, and a place for the patient and a witness to sign at the bottom. Ian had filled out his sections in advance.

"Any questions for the doctor?" the interpreter asked in Creole. Janel closed his eyes and shook his head briskly back and forth once without saying anything. It was a gesture I'd now seen many times.

Ian took a pen from his white coat pocket, clicked it, and placed it on the table next to the consent form. Janel didn't look down at the piece of paper. It was in English, which he couldn't speak or read. The Creole interpreter translated the form out loud for him. He continued to stare straight ahead. Was he scared? Determined in the face of fear? Did he even understand what this whole ritual was about?

"This paper says you understand the risks and benefits of surgery and wish to proceed," the interpreter said in Creole. "You can sign it if you agree."

Janel repeated the previous gesture, simultaneously closing his eyes and shaking his head back and forth once, then looking straight ahead again.

A confused silence settled over the room.

Brows furrowed.

After a few moments, Hermide finally spoke.

"You need to sign the form, *cheri*," she said to him softly and sweetly from across the table. "You need to sign the form so the doctors can do the operation and cure you."

Janel didn't react.

"You want to sign it?" Hermide asked, leaning forward toward him.

Another closed-eyed quick shake of his head. No.

I was seated behind Janel and off to the left, forming the third point in a triangle that included him and Ian. All eyes shifted back and forth from Janel to each other to me. My heart began to beat hard in my chest. Had he changed his mind? Or had he not really understood until now and had only just come to understand what was happening? What if after all this he just didn't want the surgery?

The silence deepened.

Usually the patient signs the form and everyone goes about their day.

I wondered if I should say something. If so, what? Should I try to tell him in Creole that he could say no, that it was okay, that he didn't have to do this if he didn't want to, that I was sorry that maybe we hadn't understood his wishes? I tried to form the phrases in Creole in my mind but couldn't seem to conjure up the words. I imagined a Hollywood-esque scene in which he'd look at me and his eyes would well up and he'd thank me and say he was just scared. He'd cry and Hermide would hug him and we'd tell him it was okay, we'd get him through this.

Or maybe this was where the story would end. Maybe he'd say he didn't want surgery, but his family had pushed him into it. He'd been afraid to say it, he'd explain, but he just wanted to stay in Haiti and leave it in God's hands. *Si Bondye vle*, as Haitians often qualified anything in the future. ("If God wants.") "When are you going home to Boston?" a colleague at HUM might ask me. "On Saturday," I'd respond. *"Samedi, si Bondye vle,"* she would say reflexively each time. ("Saturday, if God wants.")

But probably if I tried to communicate with Janel he'd just stare at me, blinking rarely. Or not even look at me. So I stayed silent. The report from our mental health colleagues in Haiti had been clear that he understood the risks and benefits of surgery and wanted to proceed. Wilner had just affirmed all this. So why was he shaking his head no?

The anesthesiologist took out her phone and started typing on it with her thumbs. All other eyes were on Janel, who continued to stare forward. I saw Ian blink a few times deliberately, dart his eyes diagonally up at the clock on the wall without turning his head, tense his jaw a bit, and then look back at Janel.

Finally, as if in slow motion, Janel lifted his right hand from his lap and tremulously moved it toward the pen. He slowly took hold of it and paused. His hand continued to shake back and forth. Ian slid the sheet of paper closer to Janel and pointed to where he was supposed to sign.

After a few moments, Janel slowly made a quivering, light, diagonal mark over the signature line. He paused there, the tip of his pen still trembling on the page.

Eyes around the table squinted at him, at the page, at the line he had just drawn.

Then Janel lifted his hand and slowly made another trembling mark. I craned my neck a bit to look over his shoulder at the consent form.

The two lines made a faint, wavy *X* that appeared to float over the signature line.

An *X*? Was this a no? Ian looked at me, and our eyes met for a brief moment. I looked across the table at Hermide, who appeared unfazed by the gesture. She was leaning toward Janel, looking at him with a beatific smile.

I heard a few heart monitor alarms and pagers going off on the ward in the distance.

Janel was still holding the pen, staring straight ahead.

Finally breaking the uncomfortable silence, I addressed Hermide. "He wrote an X," I half asked, half said. My mouth felt dry, and I swallowed hard and cleared my throat. "Is this a no?"

"No, he signed it," she replied casually. "You see, in Haiti, if people can't write their names, they will just write an X when they need to sign something." She drew an X in the air with her index finger. "So he did that." She shrugged.

A few relieved exhalations punctured the silence, as if everyone had been holding their breath. Time began moving forward again. People started gathering their belongings.

"Thanks, everyone," Ian said, taking the form, folding it, and placing it in his white coat pocket as he stood up.

The staff began chatting as Janel's nurse wheeled him out of the room. Others filed out after him.

I sat frozen in my seat, trying to make sense of what had just happened. Why had Janel shaken his head no moments before? Had it been to signal that he didn't want to sign or just that he couldn't sign? And the X . . . ?

I saw Ian leaving the room and jumped up from my chair to catch up to him in the hallway.

"Thanks so much for taking this on," I said, looking up at him.

"Thanks for involving me," he replied. "It's a huge case." He looked above me for a moment, then back at me. "We'll proceed with an infratentorial supracerebellar approach to get at the fourth ventricular component," he explained, putting one palm on top of the other and opening them at the wrist with his fingertips touching to demonstrate the space between the roof of tissue over the cerebellum (the tentorium) and the top of the cerebellum itself. He became more animated as he described the details of the operation. "I'm hoping that the upper components of the tumor will then fall into the field so we can debulk those as well." He moved his loosely cupped right hand downward and toward himself as if gently pulling an apple off a tree. "But he may need a second approach in a separate surgery."

I wondered what he was seeing in his mind as he described all of this. He had delayed surgery from the date we had initially planned, saying he needed a few days to strategize. How did the two-dimensional black-and-white MRI pictures translate into vivid three-dimensional full-color maps in his mind? And how did he use those maps to imagine his way to and through some of the most delicate areas of the brain in what would likely be a daylong surgery, or now perhaps two daylong surgeries?

"I'll keep you posted on everything," he said. "It's a fascinating case. Thanks again for involving me."

"Thank you," I said. We shook hands and then he walked past me down the hall with determined, swift, large strides—a surgeon's gait.

I went to the elevators and pushed the DOWN button. I replayed the meeting in my mind as I waited.

An X!? I shook my head, took a deep breath, puffed out my cheeks, and blew the air out in a long sigh. It was a decompression habit I had picked up sometime during my residency.

The elevator doors opened. I entered and pressed 1 for the lobby. I was alone. The doors closed, and the elevator began its slow descent.

Of course, from the medical perspective, Janel needed the surgery. Nobody would argue that. The HUM mental health team report was clear with respect to his understanding, his wishes, and his desire to have Wilner speak on his behalf. And Wilner had told us that Janel and his family would want whatever he needed to try to treat his tumor, acknowledging the risks. But Janel had made no outward sign of any of this to anyone since his arrival in Boston. He hadn't really made any outward signs at all except one smile when a young woman put on a romantic film, and then this *X*. An *X* over the signature line to his surgical consent form!

But Hermide had said it was just him signing his name, as simple as that.

As the elevator descended, I noticed I was still shaking my head. "X marks the spot," I murmured out loud to nobody and tried to force a laugh.

Except here the X meant, "Yes, you may slice open the back of my head and operate on my brain. I may have a stroke. I may have a seizure. I may be more disabled than I am now. I may even die. I understand. Go ahead."

At least that's how we interpreted it. The elevator doors opened, and I stepped out into the bright, bustling hospital lobby.

I hoped that was what he had meant.

"*Si Bondye vle,*" he might have added. If God wants.

8

Before dawn, Janel was wheeled on a gurney through swinging double doors into the operating room.

He was put under by an anesthesiologist, who then passed various lines, catheters, and tubes into his arteries, veins, lungs, and bladder to support and monitor him during the surgery.

His head was shaved and scrubbed with a dark brown iodine solution by the operating room nurses.

His limp, sedated body was lifted by the team into a seated position with his face down and arms out to the sides so Ian could approach Janel's tumor from the back of his head. Tethered by the lines and tubes coming out of his mouth, arms, and penis, he looked as if he were descending toward the floor by parachute.

His shaven head was fixed into position with a Mayfield three-point head holder—a vice with two points on one side and one on the other—to ensure there would be no movement while Ian performed a procedure requiring millimeter precision. As the vice was tightened through Janel's scalp into his skull, tiny rivulets of blood emerged around the sharp points and trickled down a few inches to his ears.

The operating room team then unfolded a tablecloth-size light blue sterile drape and laid it gently over Janel's entire body. The paper-thin drape had a square plastic window, which they positioned over the back of his head.

Ian entered backward through the swinging doors of the operating room, his arms in front of him with his elbows bent. Droplets of

water dripped from his hands, which he had spent the last several minutes washing with sterilizing soap. He was dressed in blue scrubs, a
blue bouffant cap (a wispy hairnet) covering his head, a blue surgical
mask covering his nose and mouth, and blue paper shoe covers over his
sneakers. Only his eyes and arms were exposed.

A masked nurse passed Ian a blue sterile towel, and he dried his
hands and forearms with it. The nurse then shook open a blue sterile
paper gown and held it up. Ian passed his arms into it but kept his
hands hidden inside the sleeves, the white cuffs covering his hands like
floppy mittens. He grabbed a cardboard tag from the front of the gown
with his mittened hand, handed the tag to the nurse, and then quickly
pirouetted so she could tie the gown closed in the back. Ian then slid
tan sterile surgical gloves over the cuffs of the gown and protruded his
hands from the sleeves into the gloves so that the gloves made a tight
seal over the cuffs.

The head nurse in the operating room paused for a time-out, a
standard, designated pause to make sure the right surgery was being
performed on the right patient. Everyone confirmed the patient's name
(Janel) and the operation to be performed (suboccipital craniotomy for
tumor resection).

Ian positioned the bright operating room light over the square plastic window of the blue drape. The operating room nurse passed him a
scalpel. Along the same line he had traced with his finger days before,
Ian made a vertical incision from Janel's occiput to midway down his
neck. Bright red blood oozed around the wake of the scalpel's path, and
Ian's assisting resident suctioned it away with a straw-size vacuum to
clear the operating field. Together they gently retracted the scalp and
the skin of the back of the neck to give access to the muscles beneath,
which they then teased apart to bring the skull into view.

Using an electric drill, Ian bored four holes into the skull, each creating a sawdust-like mound that his assisting resident dampened with
sterile water and wiped away with gauze. The four holes outlined a
Post-it-size square. Ian connected the dots with a small saw and gently

lifted out the swatch of bone, revealing the blood-streaked tan dura mater beneath. Meaning "tough mother" in Latin, the dura mater is a thick protective outer covering of the brain.

At this point, Ian brought a microscope over the operating field, which magnified his hands to cartoon proportions. Under the microscope, he sliced opened the dura mater to bring the cerebellum into view, its intricate fern-like surface pulsating with each heartbeat. A fist-size structure that sits at the back and bottom of the brain, the cerebellum contains as many neurons as the whole rest of the brain, which it uses to control and coordinate movements. It was the tumor's distortion of this structure that we thought had led to Janel's tremulousness and inability to walk.

The cerebellum is draped from above by a flap of dura mater called the tentorium, which provides a tent over it, as the name suggests. The tentorium is the structure that Ian had mimicked with his top hand in the palm-to-palm demonstration of his surgical approach after the meeting a few days earlier.

Between the cerebellum and its protective tent was a bulging, thin, gray membrane: the tumor's posterior, fluid-filled, cystic component. Ian pierced it. Clear fluid spilled out, which his assistant suctioned away. Peering into the ventricular system—the hollow cavities at the center of the brain—Ian got his first glimpse of the core of the tumor, a firm, rubbery, gray mass encasing large veins (which, if damaged, could lead to fatal bleeding) and extending upward and outward to the border of the thalamus (which, if damaged, could lead to coma).

Bit by grain-of-salt-size bit, Ian patiently dissected fragments of the tumor, alternating between various tools: scalpel, bipolar (electrified tweezers that burn the tumor), and Cavitron ultrasonic surgical aspirator (CUSA, for short, which liquefies the tumor and slurps out the liquefied fragments). He sent samples of tumor tissue to the pathology lab.

Despite hours of careful microsurgery, a large portion of the tumor still remained out of reach, failing to fall into the operative field as Ian had hoped. He tried a different approach, gently lifting the back of the brain off the top of the tentorium and passing between them. But the tumor's deepest components still remained inaccessible.

"I did not feel at this point that I was going to be successful at bringing more tumor down, and I felt that I had maximized the tumor we could resect from this one exposure," Ian would later transcribe in his operative report. Janel would need a second surgery.

Ian and his team closed the dura mater by sewing in a synthetic patch. Using titanium plates and screws, they reattached the Post-it-size piece of bone they'd removed earlier in the operation. Then, as if closing a successive series of curtains on this nearly ten-hour performance, they sewed together the muscle, the tissues beneath the scalp, and the scalp itself. Finally, they covered the surgical site with a large white gauze bandage.

I had been seeing patients in the hospital all day, nervously awaiting news from Ian. The only message I had received was an email from one of the pathologists around 1 p.m. He had written that he had received a specimen from the operating room, but despite having four expert colleagues examine it under the microscope with him, none of them could tell what type of tumor it was. The tissue would require further testing to make a diagnosis.

Just after 3 p.m., I received an email from Ian:

> We are finishing up—I couldn't get it all from the posterior approach that we adopted. It's a very firm (read, "miserable!") tumor and so I resected everything I could get from that approach. We went supracerebellar infratentorial and also supratentorial (occipital transtentorial), but it's such a firm tumor that I will have to approach the upper and lateral portions in a separate case.

I think everything went well. Path has no idea what this is.
It'll be a long wake up, but when we get a sense of how he is
doing, will let you know.

My emotions were mixed. I was relieved that the surgery had gone
well. But it was concerning that Janel would need a second surgery and
we had no idea what type of tumor it was. And how long would the
"long wake up" take?

Months before I had found out about Janel, Nina and I had planned
our honeymoon in Cambodia and Vietnam for this period. Our work
schedules hadn't overlapped for a trip just after our summer wedding,
so we had strategically planned an escape from the Boston winter instead. I was about to leave in thirty-six hours and was feeling guilty
about it. Even after I'd first learned about Janel in September, I hadn't
imagined it would take over three months to get him to Boston. And
once we got him to Boston, I hadn't anticipated that it would be a week
before surgery, let alone that he would need a second surgery. Anne,
Michelle, and Hermide assured me that I deserved a vacation. I wasn't
directly contributing to Janel's treatment at this point anyway. Still, it
felt irresponsible to go away for two weeks at such a critical juncture in
his care. Would the long wake up mean he wouldn't even be awake yet
when I left?

The morning after the surgery, I went to see Janel in the neurology intensive care unit (neuro-ICU). On the ninth floor of Brigham's
towers, the neuro-ICU is shaped in an arc, a common ICU design allowing medical staff to see all patients and their monitors from a central station. ICUs care for the sickest patients in the hospital. In the
neuro-ICU, this includes patients with massive strokes or brain hemorrhages, uncontrollable seizures, severe head trauma, and patients
who have undergone long and complex brain surgeries like Janel's.

Making my way along the arc, I spotted Janel. His head was wrapped
in a turban of tight white gauze. He lay motionless, his eyes closed,

lines and tubes protruding from nearly every orifice and limb: a drain catheter taped to the side of his head and connected to a bedside pressure gauge attached to a metal pole; a tangle of wires running from his scalp to a computer screen, which displayed the countless squiggly lines of his brain waves; a breathing tube protruding from his mouth connected to a ventilator (breathing machine); IVs pouring medications into his arms from clear plastic pouches hanging on IV poles; monitors attached to his arms tracking his heart rate, oxygen, and blood pressure; and tubes emerging from beneath his blue-and-white checkered hospital gown draining his bladder and rectum of urine and stool.

The only sound in the room was the rhythmic whoosh of the ventilator, a sound that always reminded me of Darth Vader's breathing—*haooooooKHssssshhhh . . . haoooKHssssshhh . . .*

When I first began my medical training, I found ICUs incredibly frightening. The patients are very sick and their care is extremely complex. All those lines and tubes generate reams of data to evaluate the function of every organ, requiring moment-to-moment vigilance, interpretation, and reaction. And then there are the mere mechanics of maneuvering in the small, crowded ICU rooms—what if I accidentally tripped on something and disconnected the breathing tube or a life-sustaining IV?

Patients sick enough to need the ICU sometimes emerge as big saves, a testament to modern medical technology. But many patients die in the ICU after a last-ditch effort to intervene in a medical emergency. And between those extremes are the patients who remain in some ambiguous limbo state—surviving but not improving enough to make it out of the ICU—leaving families in the challenging position of deciding whether to keep going or let go without a clear prognosis from the medical team. Over time, I had become more comfortable assessing patients in these critically ill states.

I approached Janel's bed.

haooooooKHssssshhhh . . . haoooKHssssshhh . . .

"Is he on any sedation?" I asked his nurse. If patients are receiving sedating medications, then their true level of consciousness can't be determined. Since sedatives to induce coma are often needed to keep patients comfortable on the ventilator, we would need to turn those off briefly to see if Janel could wake up and respond.

"No, he's been off since midnight," his nurse replied. This meant that if I couldn't wake Janel up, it was due to his brain, not the effect of any medications being given to him.

I turned back to Janel.

haoooooooKHssssshhhh . . . haoooKHssssshhh . . .

"Janel," I said just loud enough to be heard over the ventilator.

No response.

haoooooooKHssssshhhh . . . haoooKHssssshhh . . .

"Janel, ouvri zye w," I said. ("Janel, open your eyes.")

No response.

haoooooooKHssssshhhh . . . haoooKHsssshhh . . .

"Ja-NEL!" I tried again, louder and closer to his face. If a patient who appears to be in a coma doesn't respond to a normal voice, the next step is to try a progressively louder voice.

No response.

haoooooooKHssssshhhh . . . haoooKHsssshhh . . .

"JANEL, OUVRI ZYE W!" I shouted. ("JANEL, OPEN YOUR EYES!")

Still no response.

If there is no response to a loud voice, we try progressively vigorous physical stimulation. I gently pushed on the middle of Janel's chest with my fingertips, saying his name again.

No response.

I pushed more deeply and moved my fingers back and forth on his chest.

Nothing.

Finally, I proceeded to what we call noxious stimulation. I made a fist, pressed my knuckles into the center of Janel's sternum, and rubbed back and forth hard enough to shake him.

haoooooooKHssssshhhh . . . haoooKHssssshhh . . .

No response to this either.

I was beginning to get concerned.

I reached over his head and gently pulled open his eyelids with my thumb and first finger, resting my palm on his forehead. His eyes were looking all the way to the left. Now I was alarmed. Deviation of the eyes can be caused by large strokes or seizures.

haoooooooKHssssshhhh . . . haoooKHssssshhh . . .

I looked up at the EEG (electroencephalogram) monitoring Janel's brain waves. Rows of undulating lines. None had the sharp, rhythmic contour of seizures.

I darted my hand toward each eye without touching it to see if he'd blink in response. He didn't. I shined a flashlight in each eye. His pupils looked about the same as before surgery, the right slightly larger than the left. Neither constricted in response to the light.

"He's got a gag when we suction him, but that's about it," his nurse said. At least one of his vital reflexes—gagging when the back of the throat is stimulated—was present.

Since patients in a coma can't hear us if we ask them to move their arms or legs (or if they somehow can hear us, they can't respond), we resort to pinching each limb to see if the patient can sense pain and move in response to it.

With my thumb and index finger, I pinched just above the fingernail of Janel's left index finger. As I applied increasing pressure, his elbow slowly began to bend to pull away from me. This meant he could feel it and he could react, the first sign of some basic neurologic function. He responded similarly when I pinched his left big toe. But in the right arm and leg, no matter how hard I pinched, there was no movement. Either he couldn't feel it or he couldn't respond.

My concern was growing. Although Ian had warned of a long wake up, there was no reason Janel should have asymmetries in his ability to react to pain unless he had suffered a complication on one side of his brain. The combination of his eyes deviating to one side and weakness on the opposite side suggested he could have had a massive stroke or brain hemorrhage. I was worried that my worst fear—that surgery could harm Janel rather than help him—appeared to have come true.

haoooooKHssssshhhh . . . haoooKHsssshhh . . .

I looked up to see one of the neuro-ICU doctors entering. "Were you able to get anything on the right?" she asked.

I shook my head no.

"We weren't either," she said matter-of-factly. "He's going for an MRI to look for a stroke or a hemorrhage."

"What do you make of the gaze deviation?" I asked.

"Doesn't look like he's seizing on EEG." She shrugged. "I guess we'll see what the MRI shows."

The neuro-ICU was a place that was very familiar to me. I had spent six weeks of long days and four weeks of long nights there as a resident. But I had taken care of the neurology patients and wasn't familiar with what to expect in the neurosurgery patients.

"Are you worried he's not waking up yet?" I asked.

"Not yet," she said. "These patients take a while to wake up after such a big surgery. Presuming his MRI is clean, we just need to give him time. Ian said he suspects he'll come around in a few days."

I went to my office to get some last-minute work finished before leaving on our honeymoon the next day while I waited for Janel's MRI results. What if he'd had a stroke during the surgery? Or a brain hemorrhage? Both were possible complications. I tried to remind myself that these were risks we had to take to attempt to help him, risks we had discussed with him and his family. I wondered how Wilner would react if Anne called him in Haiti to explain that Janel had suffered a complication. I imagined it would be with calm acceptance, with faith that Janel would recover.

When the MRI was available to review, I went first to the images that would reveal strokes and quickly scrolled through. Normal: no stroke. I then scrolled through the sequences that would display bleeding. Normal: no hemorrhage. I realized I had been holding my breath and slowly released it.

Now that the most worrisome possibilities were off the table, I looked more closely at the brain stem and cerebellum, the structures at the base of the brain where Ian had performed the surgery. These structures had been horribly distorted on Janel's original scan. But now that the tumor was partially removed, they had expanded nearly back to their normal shapes. "Wow," I said, smiling. The brain stem and cerebellum had likely been compressed by this tumor for years. Yet what resilience! There was no reason Janel shouldn't wake up, at least not according to the scan. I tried to tell myself it was okay to go on vacation—there was nothing I could do in Boston but watch and wait.

As Nina and I arrived at the airport the next morning, I received a text message from Ian.

> Our man better today, possible extubation—moving right better too.

Thanks to Anne's and Michelle's emails while I was away, I followed Janel's daily progress. Two days after surgery, he was able to breathe on his own and came off the ventilator (extubation). Three days after surgery, he was able to sit up on his own. And four days after surgery, he began eating and talking a bit.

Trying to balance enjoying our honeymoon and keeping up-to-date with what was happening with Janel was easier than I had anticipated, since we were twelve hours ahead of Boston time. Each morning I could check my email and find out what had happened the previous day. But then I could relax for the rest of the day knowing it was nighttime in Boston, when I was unlikely to get any texts or emails.

A week after surgery, Anne wrote to me excitedly that Janel was more and more talkative and even reached out and shook her hand.

He looked the best anyone had seen him since he arrived in Boston. I was thrilled and wrote back thanking her for this encouraging news. She told me to stop checking my email and enjoy my honeymoon. But Nina and I both knew that being unplugged and wondering about what was happening would have been more nerve-wracking for me than just staying connected.

On the day of the second surgery, ten days after the first, Ian wrote to me:

> I am hoping we can clean him out today. It's such a large and firm mass that there is a chance that one approach today may not do it either. If he lived here, I would let him recover for a few weeks and bring him back for whatever he needed, if he needed it. I am not sure if we have that luxury with him?

I saw the email had been sent just a half hour before I read it—early morning before surgery in Boston, early evening before dinner on one of the last days of our trip to Vietnam. If Ian thought Janel needed a few weeks more before the second operation, there was no rush, so I wrote back immediately to let him know that we had time.

There was no reply by the time we came back from dinner to our hotel. Janel was already in the operating room. I would have to wait until the next morning for an update.

Whereas in the first surgery Janel was seated and facing downward, for the second he was placed on his back with his chin directed toward his chest, as if he were floating at the surface of a lake. Ian would be approaching the tumor from the top of his head this time rather than from the back, as he had done in the first operation.

After all of the preparations were made, Ian slowly traced his scalpel in an arc from just above Janel's left ear to just above his right. His assisting resident followed the scalpel with white gauze that turned maroon as he mopped up the blood that emerged. They then worked together to gently tease the scalp away from the skull with the blunt end of the scalpel. With the scalp loosened from the skull, they carefully peeled Janel's forehead over his eyes, as if pulling off a Halloween mask. Then they peeled back the scalp at his hairline, exposing a wide crescent of skull, the white of the bone tinged with blood from the undersurface of the scalp.

Ian used a small saw to trace the edges of this crescent of skull, lifted out the piece of bone, and set the piece aside in a basin of sterile water. Then he brought the operative microscope into place over the left side of Janel's head.

He sliced a flap in the dura mater and opened it upward like an eyelid to reveal the brain beneath, blood-streaked, pink-tan, and glistening, sinuous arteries and veins covering it like a system of small red and blue streams.

The brain is divided into the left and right hemispheres. Ian gently spread the two hemispheres an inch apart and placed two sterile cotton balls between them to keep them slightly separated. This allowed him to look directly down on the smooth white bundle called the corpus callosum, a thick bridge of fibers that connects the two hemispheres. He carefully sliced through it.

Through this incision, Ian could see the fluid-filled spaces of the ventricles beneath. He was now within striking distance of the gray, firm mass of tumor that had eluded him in the first surgery.

Now began the debulking process—attempting to get as much tumor bulk out as possible without damaging any normal tissue. Ian's main concern was the delicate, deep veins encased by the tumor. Over several hours, Ian liquefied and suctioned off small bits of the mass. Piece by minuscule piece, he eventually carved the left side of the tumor to a small enough size that he could appreciate its relationship to one of the veins beneath it. Ian proceeded even more slowly and cautiously at this stage, liquefying and suctioning until there was just a small rind of

tumor attached to the vein. He left it there to avoid injuring the important blood vessel.

Then he opened a flap in the dura mater on the right side and spent
the next few hours debulking the right side of the tumor, performing a
mirror image of the operation he had just completed on the left. Again,
he left a tiny rind of tumor attached to the vein on that side to prevent
damage to it.

In his characteristically understated operative report, Ian would
later write, "We were satisfied with a very significant resection here."
From the size of a lemon to two small slivers was a very significant
resection indeed. But just as important as the amount of tumor he had
removed was his judiciousness in knowing how much to leave behind.
"The best neurosurgeons are the ones who know when to stop," my
neurology mentor Marty Samuels once opined. By pursuing an aggressively maximal resection while minimizing the potential for complications, Ian is indeed one of the best neurosurgeons.

After stitching the dura back together and reattaching the crescent
of bone with titanium plates and screws, Ian and his assisting resident
unfurled the flaps of scalp they had pulled apart, lined the edges up
carefully, and sewed them back together with black sutures.

By the time I woke up the next morning in Vietnam (evening in Boston), I had this update from Ian by email:

> We just finished—everything went very well. I think we have
> a very significant resection from this different trajectory. We
> will let him recover for a couple of days and then likely put a
> shunt in if I can't wean his drain.

I was relieved to hear that the surgery was successful but worried
about the possibility of Janel needing a shunt.

A shunt is a system of plastic and rubber tubing with one end placed in the brain's ventricles, the other in the abdomen, and the tubing between them tunneled under the skin of the chest. This allows for elevated pressure in the ventricles to be relieved by draining some of their excess fluid into the abdomen.

Implanting a shunt is a relatively minor neurosurgical procedure, but having a plastic and rubber device connecting the brain and abdomen can lead to complications at any time. A shunt can become infected. It can develop mechanical malfunction, causing it to stop working, leading to a dangerous rise in intracranial pressure. Both complications require surgery to repair or replace the shunt. Such surgeries could be easily performed in the US. But if Janel were to suffer any of these complications after his return to Haiti, there was no guarantee we would be able to get him treated in time, if at all.

I remembered seeing a woman in rural Haiti who brought her baby to the hospital covered in a gray blanket. She pulled back the top of the blanket to reveal an enormous, bulbous, alien-like head with a huge protuberant forehead dwarfing a tiny face below it. Large tortuous veins stood out over the entire head like hanging vines. The shiny scalp was stretched so taut over the expanded skull that it looked as if it could burst. The infant was comatose.

She told us the baby had gotten a shunt at birth, several months prior. We told her that the shunt didn't appear to be working and that it needed to be evaluated and perhaps repaired or replaced immediately. She said she had gone back to the hospital where the baby had gotten the shunt but was refused further treatment since she couldn't pay. She had spent all of her family's money on the first shunt surgery.

I had seen several children in Haiti who had undergone a shunt procedure in infancy for congenital hydrocephalus, had developed a shunt complication later in childhood, and then were unable to find or afford another surgery to address the issue. This could be fatal.

I wrote to Ian expressing my concerns about dealing with a shunt in Haiti and asked him if there were any alternatives. His reply:

> I think he will need a shunt. I suspect he has had elevated
> intracranial pressure for some time. We will try to wean his
> drain after today's surgery, but he may need it.

The drain he was referring to was a catheter that ran from the ventricles of Janel's brain to an external pressure monitor through a small hole drilled in the skull. It had been placed in the operating room and left in after surgery to serve as a temporary shunt while the brain recovered from surgery. Weaning the drain meant clamping its outflow to observe the result. If the pressure remained normal with the drain clamped, it could be removed. If the pressure rose, Janel could need a more permanent solution: a shunt.

Our hope was that with the tumor removed, the ventricles would return to their normal size, and the flow of cerebrospinal fluid would return to its normal dynamics. Time would tell.

Two days later, when Nina and I were at the airport, waiting to fly home, I got an email update from Ian.

> Janel is coming around slowly, similar to his last wake up.
> He is awake, saying a few things, following commands with
> his left side reliably, beginning to move the right side weakly.
> I suspect he will come around in time.
>
> Anyway, we have to give this young man time to recover.
>
> I really appreciate that you involved me here.

Encouraged by Ian's message, I was eager to see Janel. After sleeping off our twenty-hour flight home to Boston, I went to the hospital the next morning.

Janel was still in the neuro-ICU. Thick black stitches ran in an ear-to-ear arc along his hairline, resembling a zipper. A thin yellow tube coming from his nose was taped to the side of his face—it was being used to feed him and passed all the way from his nose to his stomach. He stared ahead, wide-eyed, blinking rarely. I said his name, but he didn't respond to my voice. He occasionally moved his arms and legs a little, but that was it. I thought once when I asked him to move his left arm he did it, but I wasn't sure if it was in response to me or if he had just moved it coincidentally at the time I had given him the instruction. He looked awful.

Later that day, I ran into Ian and asked him how he thought Janel was doing. He could see I was worried. "He'll come around," he said with casual confidence. "Give him some time."

Morning after morning over that week, I continued to visit Janel's bedside before I started my workday. The ear-to-ear incision began to look more like an early scar and less like a fresh wound. He appeared awake but not clearly alert. His eyes were always wide open, staring forward, but it was unclear if he was seeing anything.

Each morning I went through the same steps: saying his name a few times (no response), shouting his name a few times (no response), trying to get him to follow some simple directions in Creole ("Stick out your tongue," "Close your eyes"—no response), poking briskly toward each eye without touching it (sometimes it looked like he blinked in response, but I was never convinced that it wasn't just a coincidental blink), and finally rubbing his sternum with my knuckles (he moved his arms and legs a little bit but didn't make any clear effort to stop me). He was unable to interact with me in any meaningful way.

I was growing concerned that Janel could become what I sometimes irreverently described as "neurosurgical success, neurological failure": the surgery had gone technically well as far as the neurosurgeons were concerned (no more tumor), but the patient was no better off—or even worse off—than before the operation.

Ian and his team tried several times to wean Janel from the drain by clamping it off to see if his brain could tolerate this. Each time, the intracranial pressure on the monitor rose dramatically and clear cerebrospinal fluid oozed from around the site where the drain entered the scalp. Janel would need a shunt. The shunt surgery would be minor compared to the first two, but it would still require another round of anesthesia, and he still hadn't woken up from the second surgery.

And so ten days after his second surgery, twenty days after his first, having never left the neuro-ICU, Janel went for his third surgery to have the shunt implanted.

———————

The pathologists puzzled over the appearance of Janel's tumor under the microscope. After performing a number of specialized tests on the tissue and analyzing its genetic makeup, they finally reached a diagnosis: a tumor of the pineal gland called a pineal parenchymal tumor of intermediate differentiation, or PPTID. I had never heard of it. The oncologist and radiation oncologist who specialized in brain tumors and who would be treating Janel had heard of it but had never seen a case.

The pineal gland is a small seed-size structure deep in the center of the brain. Its name comes from its resemblance to a miniature pine cone. Seventeenth-century philosopher René Descartes thought the pineal gland was the seat of the soul. Some spiritual traditions believe it is the anatomical correlate of the mystical third eye. Neurologists don't give it much thought. It calcifies with age, and this calcium provides a bright anatomical landmark on CT scans. It occasionally develops benign cysts that rarely cause clinical effects. It produces melatonin, a chemical involved in the sleep–wake cycle, but tumors of the gland (or surgery to treat them) do not appear to have any significant effect on sleep. Pineal tumors are rare, accounting for less than one percent of all brain tumors.

Brain tumors are graded on a scale of 1 to 4 based on how aggressive they appear under the microscope: 1 is the most benign, 4 is the most malignant. Grade 1 pineal tumors are called pineocytomas, and grade

4 tumors are called pineoblastomas. Intermediate tumors considered grade 2 or grade 3 are so uncommon that they didn't earn a succinct name, so they are classified as PPTIDs.

For the relatively benign pineocytomas, surgery is often enough to fully treat the tumor, with radiation added if the tumor cannot be fully removed. For the malignant pineoblastomas, surgery, radiation, and chemotherapy are needed to reduce the risk of recurrence. As for PPTIDs, they are so rare that there is hardly any scientific literature on how to treat them.

The pathologists classified Janel's tumor as grade 3. This suggested it was highly aggressive. But with so few reported cases, it was unclear how aggressively to treat it. The oncologist and radiation oncologist at Brigham who would be treating Janel wrote to other brain tumor experts around the country to discuss his case. These experts recommended that we err on the side of being maximally aggressive, treating Janel's tumor as we would treat a pineoblastoma, the most malignant pineal tumor. This would require eight months of intensive treatment: two months of daily brain radiation and chemotherapy, followed by three days of chemotherapy per month for the next six months.

Janel was going to need to spend nearly a year in Boston. Nothing seemed to be going as planned.

It was the end of January, one week after the shunt operation, two weeks after the second surgery, and almost a month since the first surgery. I continued to check on Janel every morning before work. He had finally made it out of the neuro-ICU and back to the tenth floor neurology ward where he had first arrived, but he still didn't seem to be able to do anything except stare and occasionally move his arms and legs. I was increasingly concerned that we'd failed on one of medicine's guiding principles: do no harm.

I trusted Ian, and I hadn't taken care of any patients after such massive neurosurgeries to know how long it took them to wake up. But

Janel looked worse than before all of his surgeries, and I was troubled that there was no explanation for why he remained in this state—at least not one that our high-tech medical tests could pick up. Janel's scans showed he hadn't had a stroke or brain hemorrhage, and EEGs (recordings of his brain waves) showed he wasn't having seizures. Still, I worried. Maybe he had suffered some microscopic damage to his thalamus during the surgery that was too small to detect on the MRI. Or maybe he had developed a condition called posterior fossa syndrome, in which patients become mute after large surgeries involving the posterior aspect of the brain, where Janel's first surgery had been. This syndrome is seen mostly after pediatric brain surgery, but I found some reports of it occurring in adults.

I wrote to Ian, asking what he thought about these possibilities and expressing my concern about how neurologically impaired Janel still appeared. He replied:

> He has excellent recovery potential, but he needs time after such extensive surgery. I do expect him to recover really well.

We all agreed that Janel needed intensive rehabilitation, involving physical therapy, occupational therapy, and speech therapy, to maximize his chance of at least some recovery. But our initial proposal to bring him to Brigham had been contingent in part on him not needing rehab, back when I had imagined him as an ambulatory college student who would walk into the hospital and then walk back out after surgery. We had proposed having him do rehab in Haiti as a last resort if needed, but now he needed eight months of chemotherapy and radiation therapy, and he was too debilitated to travel to Haiti in the state he was in. What I had perceived as mere logistical bureaucratic hurdles to be surmounted when advocating for Janel's care I now saw as legitimate major challenges I had been naïve not to consider more carefully. I was starting to feel like I had bitten off more than I could chew.

The cost estimate we received for a stay in a rehab facility in Boston was two thousand dollars per day, not including daily ambulance transportation back and forth to Brigham for chemotherapy and radiation. The hospital costs had already exceeded the initial estimate since Janel had needed three surgeries rather than one and had spent a month in the neuro-ICU, and we hadn't even started chemotherapy and radiation yet. The Ray Tye Medical Aid Foundation had increased its contribution to support the additional surgeries, but we didn't have any other sources of funding for the non-surgical aspects of his care.

The Brigham social worker involved in Janel's care had been trying to find a rehab center willing to provide free care for Janel for a few weeks, but she wasn't having much luck. She worried that part of the reason was a recent newspaper story describing a Haitian patient who had come to Boston for surgery after the earthquake and had been at a local rehab center ever since—for over four years. She thought this might have made local facilities wary of taking on another complex patient from Haiti.

Fortunately, our social worker was able to procure a hospital bed, wheelchair, walker, and bedside commode for Janel to use at Hermide's house. Michelle and I thought we could find a local physical therapist willing to do a few home visits. I felt horrible that we were offering Janel a better-than-nothing approach to his recovery rather than the ideal level of care he needed and deserved, but we didn't seem to have another option.

———————

Janel didn't react as I entered his hospital room during a quick lunch break between my morning and afternoon clinics. He was turned on his right side, facing the doorway to his room, his wide-open eyes gazing vacantly into nowhere. A daytime talk show played silently on the television across from his bed, the volume muted. The flickering light from the TV varied the shadows on his face. A light snow fell outside his tenth-floor window behind him. Gusts of wind between the hospital's towers occasionally sent the snow blowing upward.

"Janel?" I asked half-heartedly. It had been a month since he'd responded meaningfully to anyone. Still, every day I tried. "Janel?"

Nothing. I watched the hypnotic upward-blowing snow for a bit until it started falling downward again—a hospital-room snow globe.

I looked back at Janel. His eyes were still fixed beyond me, looking through the open door.

"*Gen nej, Janel,*" I said, more to myself than to him. ("It's snowing, Janel.")

No reaction.

"Ja-*nel!*" I tried once more, slightly louder. I got no response and walked over to the sink to wash my hands and go back to work, my daily ritual complete. While I was washing my hands, I thought I heard him say "*Wi*" behind me.

I turned around. Janel was still lying on his right side, staring out the door, expressionless. Had he just spoken? Wishful thinking—I had probably heard some other sound from the hallway and imagined it was him. I went back to washing my hands.

I was about to walk out of his room but decided to try one more time to interact with him. I went back to his bed and leaned closer to him. "*Janel, kouman ou ye?*" ("How are you?")

He blinked twice, slowly. Still gazing vacantly beyond me, he softly, hoarsely squeaked out, "*Pa pi mal, no.*" ("Not too bad, no.")

He was talking! I couldn't believe it. It was the first sign of higher brain function he had demonstrated in over a month.

"*Janel, leve bra ou nan lè,*" I asked, looking for more evidence that he was in there. ("Janel, lift up your arms.")

He stared at me. Maybe I was asking too much, but I asked again anyway. "*Janel, ale, an nou leve bra ou!*" ("Janel, come on, lift your arms!")

After a few seconds, he slowly raised his arms off the bed, then slowly placed them back down. They didn't shake.

I beamed. Ian had said that Janel would "come around," and Janel's scans had looked fine, but seeing him lie unresponsive for weeks had been disheartening. It had become hard to imagine him waking up after that. But here he was, finally beginning to come around.

"Yes!" I said a bit too loud for the hospital setting, unable to stop smiling.

Janel's nurse entered the room. "He pulled out his NG tube last night," she said. The NG (nasogastric) tube is the feeding tube that passes up the nose, down the throat, and into the stomach. They are uncomfortable, and it's not uncommon for patients to pull them out.

"That's a good sign," I said, still smiling. "Sounds like some purposeful movement!"

"He actually took in 300 cc by mouth yesterday with a lot of encouragement," she said.

"That's amazing news!" I said excitedly. Three hundred cubic centimeters is only about one cup. Not much caloric intake for a whole day. But the fact that he was awake enough to eat at all seemed like enormous progress worthy of celebration.

With each passing day, Janel spoke and ate a little more. When two physical therapists helped him stand and held him up on either side, he was able to take a few small steps. It was beginning to look like he was going to have a miraculous recovery beyond anything I could have hoped for after his discouraging course up to that point.

Highlighting Janel's dramatic improvement, our social worker was able to negotiate two weeks of free rehab for him at a local facility. When the ambulance came to transport Janel to the rehabilitation center, it was the first time he had been outside of Brigham since his arrival six weeks prior.

9

The rehab facility that accepted Janel reminded me of the nursing home where my mom had worked as a nurse when I was a child—fluorescent lighting and linoleum floors, the acrid odor of Lysol competing with the pungent smell of urine, the muted murmuring of countless televisions tuned to stations the patients hadn't chosen. It wasn't the nicest facility in the area, but we were grateful for two weeks of free rehabilitation for Janel.

With hours of daily physical therapy, he began to make small strides. His coordination improved so that he could eat on his own. His balance improved enough that he could walk the length of his room with his nurse and physical therapist supporting him. He still didn't speak much, at least not with any of us. But when we arranged a call between Janel and his mother in Haiti, he was more talkative than we had ever seen him.

Janel's mother didn't have a phone, so we had asked Wilner to visit her so Janel could speak to her on Wilner's phone. Janel kept telling his mom that he had a fever, but there was no evidence of this in his chart, and his nurses said he hadn't had one. Sometimes "having a fever" is used as an expression in Creole to simply mean "feeling ill," and it would certainly be normal to feel ill after three brain surgeries in the preceding month and a half. But did Janel really understand what had happened to him and the aggressive chemotherapy and radiation that lay ahead? I wasn't sure.

As the date of Janel's discharge from rehab to Hermide's house approached, the team at Brigham began planning for his chemotherapy and radiation. One of the Brigham oncology nurses called the staff at Janel's rehab to see how he was progressing. Then she sent me and her team a very concerned email:

> I understand that Janel is to be discharged to Hermide's home tomorrow. I spoke with the rehab nurse, and active issues continue. He is non-ambulatory, non-verbal, incontinent, impulsive, fall risk . . . Janel appears very compromised coming in for a very aggressive treatment with limited supports.

Another Brigham oncology nurse on the team replied:

> How can he be discharged?? That is concerning.

The oncologist who would be supervising Janel's treatment chimed in:

> I agree. Concerned that Janel is headed towards failure. He is requiring more care than a single person can provide.

Hermide visited Janel at rehab frequently, and either Anne or I had spoken with her nearly every day. She hadn't expressed any concerns about caring for Janel. Was she underestimating the challenges or was the oncology staff underestimating her ability to care for him? I suspected the latter.

Hermide wasn't alone. She had several other women living with her, all former patients from Haiti who had stayed to help her care for others. And Hermide had housed countless children and adults from Haiti for medical treatment in her home over the years.

Anne and I called her to see if she had any concerns. Just one, she said. At home, she felt she and the women living with her could get

Janel loaded into her car. But they wouldn't all be able to travel with her and Janel to Brigham every day. She just wanted to make sure that when she arrived at Brigham, someone would be able to help her get Janel out of the car and into a wheelchair. We reassured her that there was always help at the hospital entrance. She felt there would be no problem with the rest—feeding and bathing him at home, supporting him through his treatment at the hospital, and anything else that might come up. We asked her if she thought we should try to bring Janel's mother from Haiti to help her. She laughed. It might be nice for him, she said, but then it would be one more person for her to take care of.

Sure, Janel's care would be challenging. But Hermide's extensive experience probably made her better prepared than most people who face caring for a family member with a severe neurological condition for what is often the first and only time. And I didn't think the worried oncology staff could imagine just how well people take care of each other at home in Haitian culture.

I remembered a patient I had seen in the emergency room in Haiti just after HUM had first opened, a frail elderly woman with thinning gray hair braided into cornrows against her scalp. She lay on a gurney in a black dress printed with purple and green flowers that hung loosely on her thin frame. She was awake, but she couldn't speak, and she didn't appear to understand anything when we spoke to her. Her head and gaze were turned all the way to the left. She occasionally moved her left arm and leg, but her right arm and leg were completely paralyzed.

She appeared to be having a massive stroke, but nobody in her family seemed alarmed. They said she had been like this for about three months. Since she was in the emergency room, I had presumed it was because of a sudden event rather than a long-standing problem. I revised my diagnosis: she wasn't having a massive stroke—she had had one three months ago.

When we asked her family why they brought her to the emergency room on that particular day if she had been like this for three months, they replied, "We heard there was a new hospital, so we wondered if you might be able to do something for her."

Unfortunately, there wasn't much we could do at that point except offer physical therapy and try to reduce her risk factors for having another stroke. Although the patient's family was disappointed that we couldn't cure her, I was struck by how well she looked.

Yes, she was paralyzed on one side and mute. But in the US, if she had been brought to the hospital while she was having a stroke that large, she would have gone to an ICU, gotten IV medications, and maybe had a breathing tube and a feeding tube placed. At her age and with such pronounced neurologic disability, her family would have probably placed her in a nursing home. From there, she might have ended up back in the hospital with pneumonia from the swallowing difficulties that can occur after a stroke, which can cause food and saliva to go down the wrong pipe into the lungs. She may have gotten blood clots in her legs or bedsores on her backside and ankles from being immobile. Or maybe her family would have said that she had lived a good life and had always said that she wouldn't want to live in a state of complete dependence on others. They would have taken her home or transferred her to a hospice facility and let her fade away.

But in Haiti, her family had no hospital to bring her to, no nursing home, no hospice. So they looked after her at home. They fed her and kept her clean and free of any complications. Where doctors and hospitals are rare, and disease and disability are common, families learn to incorporate these aspects of the human condition into their daily lives. They take extraordinary care of each other.

Before I could reply to the oncology team to try to allay their anxieties, the email chain multiplied with additional concerns. How would Janel handle becoming very ill with the chemotherapy, which could cause severe nausea and vomiting? Would he be able to lie still on the radiation table with his head confined by a bolted-down form-fitting face mask? How would the hospital staff communicate with him since not only did he not speak English but he hardly ever spoke at all?

Although these were all reasonable concerns, I didn't understand why they should apply to Janel any more than to any other brain tumor patient the staff had treated. Hadn't they worked with numerous families who had challenges coping with a loved one's brain tumor and understanding the complexities of the medical system? And hadn't they cared for countless patients whose brain tumors made them confused, agitated, or otherwise difficult to communicate with while undergoing treatment?

I replied to the worried staff, describing Hermide's extensive experience, highlighting the practical point that she would not be caring for Janel alone, and expressing our confidence in her ability to care for him.

The radiation oncologist who would be treating Janel replied immediately:

> I have been so impressed with her—I am amazed that people like her exist in this world. We wouldn't be able to do this treatment without her.

The email chain quieted down.

Still, an oncology social worker met with Hermide to discuss how difficult she anticipated it would be for Hermide to take care of Janel at home. Hermide told the social worker that caring was her life's calling. It was the life she grew up with in Haiti, where her mother often cared for people who came down from the mountains to visit and receive food. "It's in my blood," she explained.

And so Janel was discharged to Hermide's home with a plan to begin chemotherapy and radiation the following week. For the first time since his arrival in Boston over two months prior, Janel slept in a home, not in a facility. He was surrounded by people who would care only for him, rather than a constantly changing cast of medical providers responsible for multiple patients at a time. Hermide and the women who lived with her cooked him Haitian food and treated him like a member of their own family. We hoped he would finally feel more comfortable. Maybe he'd even begin to talk with us.

For the first few days at Hermide's, Janel mostly slept, waking up only to eat. Though he had made some progress feeding himself and walking at rehab, he needed total assistance at meals and to get out of bed. He didn't look at his food when he ate and didn't look at his feet when he walked. He mostly communicated with Hermide through gestures. He shook his head no and raised his hand as a stop signal—for example, for any beverage aside from Pepsi. He sometimes held his head in his hands, which Hermide interpreted as meaning he had a headache, because once during this gesture he said to her that he couldn't bend his head "because he felt like blood was running out of it."

When Janel finally began to speak more, he seemed very confused. He said things like "I have to feed the cow," "I'm getting tired carrying all this wood," and "Stop hitting me with that rock. I'm just trying to get the water." Was he hallucinating or was his brain finally lurching into gear, flooding with disorganized thoughts and memories from the past few years? It wasn't clear.

The days were manageable, but the nights became battles. Janel wet the bed several times between midnight and dawn. We weren't sure if he was truly incontinent or simply went when he needed to since he had likely become accustomed to being unable to walk to the bathroom. Hermide and the women who lived with her had plenty of experience with sick kids wetting the bed, but Janel was different. He fought them. Dodging Janel's punching and kicking as she tried to undress him, get him to the bathroom to wash him, and change his sheets, Hermide told us she needed to "call on the blood of Jesus" to make it through each night.

Maybe I had brushed off the oncology staff's concerns prematurely. And maybe Hermide hadn't realized just how difficult Janel's care would be.

Hermide wrote to Anne, Michelle, and me:

You mentioned earlier that it could be possible to obtain
a visa for Janel's mother. I think this is a great idea, even a
necessity. Given the severity of the treatment, the expected
side effects, and where he is emotionally and physically,
Janel's mother can be an important factor in his recovery.
They understand each other and can communicate better.
We can do our very best, but there is nothing like the love
of a mother when one is in pain. If possible, please try to get
the visa.

We offered to try. But like Janel, his mother had no passport and no
birth certificate, so this could take months.

Somehow, in spite of all this, Hermide and the three women who
lived with her managed to get Janel to Brigham for his first days of
chemotherapy and radiation. Although the mornings were not as
chaotic as the nights, they were difficult too. Janel required a lot of encouragement and effort to get out of bed, into a wheelchair, and ultimately into the car. But Hermide persevered.

Once Janel was at the hospital, he cooperated fully. He didn't speak,
but he didn't fight either. He didn't get sick from chemotherapy, and he
remained perfectly still during his radiation treatments.

On the fourth day of treatment, Hermide went to get Janel out of
bed in the morning as she had the prior three days. He refused. First
he remained curled up in bed, not responding to her requests to wake
up. Then he pulled the covers over his head. She thought he was being
playful, but he continued to refuse to get up. When she tried to gently
guide him out of bed, he grabbed onto the bedposts. Finally, Hermide
and her helpers managed to wrestle Janel into the wheelchair. But when
they arrived at the doorway to leave the house, he splayed his legs and
pressed his feet against the outer parts of the door so they couldn't get
him through.

Hermide called me. I was working in the clinic and called her back
in between patients.

"Why do you think he's doing this?" I asked. "Did the treatment make him sick?"

"I don't know why," she said, sounding exhausted and exasperated. "Only God knows!"

"You got him into the car the last three days," I said. "Do you think you can get him to go if you keep encouraging him? It's not good to interrupt the treatment."

"Oh, I have *tried*!" she said, her normally calm, soothing voice becoming more animated, the wide-ranging lilt of her Creole accent becoming more prominent than usual. "If I force him, he might jump out of the car!" she said. "I can't risk it! Can't we just admit him back into the hospital?!"

"Well he needs daily treatment for six weeks, so that would be difficult," I replied, unsure of how to help her. "Maybe we should just take the day off and try again tomorrow?"

"I will try again tomorrow *si Bondye vle*," she said ("if God wants")— but she didn't sound happy about it.

As soon as we hung up, I called Anne to brainstorm. Maybe an external urinary catheter at night would help address the incontinence problem, and if Janel wasn't waking up all night after wetting the bed, maybe he'd be more amenable to waking up in the morning. We thought we could get a catheter from the hospital.

"Let's just try again tomorrow," Anne said. "Maybe today was a one-off thing."

Unfortunately, it wasn't. The next day was exactly the same. So was the next. The oncology team was getting frustrated, understandably so. They had to set up each day to prepare for Janel's treatment and were concerned that erratic dosing of radiation and chemotherapy would be ineffective in treating his tumor. I was beginning to realize that I had been naïvely optimistic when I had tried to reassure them that everything would work out fine in spite of their concerns.

We decided to cancel the rest of the week's treatments and regroup.

When Anne went to visit Janel at Hermide's, she found him awake in bed. He didn't speak but would nod yes and no to questions, though not always logically—he nodded yes when she asked him if he was in Haiti. Anne took out her phone and showed Janel a picture of his mother that one of our colleagues in Haiti had sent her. His normal expressionless stare brightened into the broad, toothy smile we had seen only once before. He grabbed the phone, clutched it to his chest, closed his eyes, and shimmied back and forth. Then his smile slowly faded back to his silent stare.

Anne asked Hermide what had changed from the week before when things seemed to be going well. She said nothing had changed. It had been just as difficult during the first few days, but she had pushed through. She just felt that she couldn't continue to strong-arm and reprimand Janel.

We asked for help from a young Haitian psychiatrist from HUM who was doing his master's in Boston. The psychiatrist was able to get more verbal interaction from Janel than we were and asked him how his hospital visits were going. Janel said they were fine and didn't mention anything about resisting them. Janel quickly tired of the psychiatrist's questions and pulled the sheet over his head. The psychiatrist encouraged him to keep going to the hospital. He said Janel gave him a soft *"Wi"* ("Yes") of agreement from underneath the sheets. The psychiatrist's interpretation was that maybe, culturally, Janel needed a male authority figure to be more firm with him. He suggested calling Wilner to hear his perspective.

Together, the psychiatrist and Hermide called Wilner, who told them that he had never seen Janel be combative, but the incontinence, minimal verbal communication, and complete dependence on others for eating and walking were similar to what he had observed when Janel lived with him. Wilner didn't understand why Janel was refusing treatment but apologized, saying he was ashamed that Janel was behaving this way. Wilner believed that Janel's behavior must be part of his disease and not what Janel would really want—he would want to be treated for his condition. Wilner encouraged us to do whatever it took to complete Janel's treatment.

Wilner spoke to Janel and asked him to promise that he would participate in his care and stop resisting the efforts of Hermide and the ladies living with her. Then Wilner told Hermide to speak to Janel with more authority in her voice.

After Janel had a few days' rest from going to the hospital, Hermide thought he was doing much better. He asked her to help him out of bed, then walked with minimal assistance downstairs and watched television with her. When Michelle visited, he greeted her with a smile and a handshake.

By the end of the weekend, we felt encouraged. We concluded that arriving at Hermide's house and starting treatment were a lot for him to adjust to all at once. Since he seemed to be settling in, Hermide felt we could try to restart treatment the following week, and she said Janel had agreed. We let the oncology team know.

Monday arrived, and since I hadn't heard anything from Hermide by the time I finished my morning clinic and took a quick break for lunch, I presumed everything was going well. But just after noon, Anne and I received an email from one of the oncology nurses that Hermide had called them to say that Janel was curled up in the fetal position and she couldn't get him out of bed.

Seconds after the email came through, my phone rang. It was Anne. "What happened?" I asked her.

"Same thing. He wouldn't get out of bed," she said.

"Did she call Wilner?" I asked.

"She did, but it was too late," she replied. "After Wilner talked to Janel on the phone for a while, Janel agreed to get out of bed and go to the hospital, but they had already missed their appointment. They're going to try to get Wilner on the phone first thing in the morning tomorrow. Let's give it one more try."

"Okay, but what are we going to do if this doesn't work?" I asked.

"I guess we'll just have to wait until we can get his mom here and see if that helps," she said.

"But that could be months," I replied, concerned that we didn't have a good plan in place.

"What else can we do?" she asked. "He needs the treatment, right?"

"True," I said. "Well, let's cross our fingers."

I pleaded with the oncology team to give Janel one more chance to get into a rhythm, explaining our new plan of having Wilner on the phone in the early morning. They kindly agreed but warned me that as Janel received more treatment, he would become sicker, and so things were only likely to get harder for him and for everyone else. Though I had pushed back against their concerns before, now I shared them.

I sat in my office the next morning trying to focus on finishing clinic notes from the previous day's patients and reviewing patient charts for my clinic that afternoon. But I kept imagining Hermide begging Janel, pushing him and pulling him, the women who lived with her wrestling him into a wheelchair. If Janel didn't like going to the hospital, this would certainly be understandable. But once he was in the hospital, he calmly cooperated with all aspects of his treatment. He didn't resist or complain about having his head tightly encased in a mask bolted to a table for radiation therapy. He barely flinched when he was stuck with IV needles. So why was he so resistant at home? Hermide treated him so lovingly and patiently, like her own child. It didn't make sense.

I thought of an old neurology riddle: "When is a patient with Parkinson's disease most likely to fall?" the professor asks. "Late in the disease?" a student answers, falling into the professor's trap. "No, after getting on the right medications!" the professor replies, in a gotcha tone. Patients who have been slowed and immobilized by Parkinson's disease for years can suddenly gain newfound fluidity and energy with the right treatment, and often overestimate their abilities. In their overeagerness, they sometimes try to move faster than their bodies are ready to, and fall.

Could it be that Janel's brain was beginning to function better after years of severe impairment, but he wasn't yet in control of his new mental faculties and not entirely aware of what he could and couldn't do? Was he confused as his brain woke up to a reality far from Haiti, with no clear memory of how he got there?

My phone was ringing. It was Hermide.

I sighed, answered, and braced for the worst.

"Doctor Aaron, we are in front of Brigham, but Janel is refusing to get out of the car!" she said, flustered. "We don't know what we can do!"

At least they had made it this far, I thought. "Which entrance are you at?" I asked.

"The main entrance," Hermide said.

"I'll be right there," I said and hung up.

I put on my winter coat and started making my way across campus, wondering how I was going to get any of my work done with Janel's care becoming nearly all-consuming. Still, I was curious to see what this whole scene looked like after hearing about it secondhand for the prior week.

Hermide was parked in front of the main entrance to the hospital with the back right car door open. Janel was sitting in the back seat next to the open door, staring forward. A hospital staff member was waiting patiently outside the car with a wheelchair.

"*Bonjou, Janel,*" I said. ("Hi, Janel.")

"*Bonjou,*" he said in his high-pitched croak after a delay, still staring straight ahead.

"*Mwen kontan we w,*" I said. ("I'm happy to see you.")

After another delay, he replied, "*Mwen menm too.*" ("Me too.")

"*W vle vini pou tretman an?*" I asked. ("Would you like to come in for your treatment?")

"*Dako,*" he said, after a pause. ("Okay.")

"*Vini,*" I said. ("Come.")

After a few seconds, he gradually turned his head to look at me.

He blinked slowly a few times.

"Ale, an nou vini," I said, reaching out my hands to him. ("Come on, let's go.")

He looked at me for a few seconds without moving. Then, slowly, he reached out his arms. I motioned to the staff member waiting with the wheelchair to come closer, and we gently stood Janel up, helped him pivot his back to the wheelchair, and guided him down into the seat.

"Mm! He listens to you!!" Hermide said from the front seat, shaking her head.

"I'm not sure why," I replied, surprised we had gotten him out of the car so easily.

"Well! Maybe because you are a man!? I don't know!" She had that angry inflection of her accent coming through again.

I let out a little laugh. "Is it really that simple?" I asked. "Well, at least we got him out of the car."

Hermide looked away and shook her head, making a *tsk* sound. I said goodbye and ran to my clinic, where I was late and had to apologize to my patients for keeping them waiting.

As usual, once he was in the hospital, Janel did fine. The radiation oncologist wrote to me that it required some effort and encouragement to get Janel onto the radiation table, but once on it, he did great, without moving or any other issues. "We cleared out all of the men—he responded very well to an all female team (not sure why, but we'll take it)," he wrote to me in an email. Janel even gave one of the nurses a high five on his way out. "He is definitely present," the nurse wrote in her treatment note for the day, "but the extent is not clear."

That afternoon, I had a break between patients in my clinic and stopped by to visit Janel while he was getting his treatment. I walked by patients bald and pale from chemotherapy sitting in rows of large green-blue reclining hospital chairs separated by tan curtains, medications running into their veins through IVs connected to clear plastic bags hanging from metal poles next to their chairs.

Hermide was sitting in a chair next to Janel. When I arrived, she used it as a chance to take a break so she could feed her parking meter and get something to eat. Janel sat quietly, his chair fully reclined, a white hospital blanket pulled up to just below his eyes, which were gently closed. They hadn't started his chemotherapy yet. A nurse came to talk to him about his treatment for that day. An interpreter translated. Janel kept his eyes closed and didn't respond.

"I'm going to need to access your port. Can you bring the blanket down?" the nurse asked him gently.

The interpreter translated.

Janel didn't respond. The nurse and I tried to gently bring down the blanket to expose his upper chest. At first he held on to the blanket, resisting. But after a moment, he let go. He'd been through this before, but the nurse talked him through it anyway.

"First I just have to clean off the area," she said. With her purple-gloved hands, she rubbed dark brown antiseptic solution in small circles over the bulge just below Janel's right clavicle.

"Okay, now a little stick," she said, bringing the needle toward him.

His eyes were open now and followed the needle's path toward his chest.

"One, two, three, little pinch!" his nurse said and plunged the needle into the port. A brief flicker of a wince flashed over Janel's face and then he closed his eyes again.

Hermide came back. "How's he doing?" she asked.

"Seems to be doing okay," I said. "How are *you* doing?" I asked her.

"We take it one day at time," she said. "God knows!"

Let's hope we can get through one day at a time for six more weeks, I thought, but didn't say. Instead, I said, *"Piti piti . . ."* ("Little by little . . .")

She smiled. "Ah, you know that proverb?"

"Piti piti, zwazo fe nich li," I said, smiling back. ("Little by little, the bird builds its nest.")

She laughed. "Oh! Your Creole is coming along!"

I told her I had to run back to my clinic, and she nodded.

"Thank you, Hermide," I said, taking her hand. "You are a true saint," I added in Creole.

She slowly shook her head no, then returned her attention to Janel.

When I turned back from the doorway to the infusion suite, I saw her looking down on him with a peaceful smile, softly stroking his head.

The next day was uneventful. So was the next. And the one after that. The nurses were taking a liking to Janel.

A nurse wrote to us:

> Just wanted to let you all know that Janel was here for treatment today. He was very resistant at first, not letting me do anything I needed to. However, after some time he eventually allowed me to do his infusion and even change his clothes because he was incontinent. I even got a smile and a "merci" as he was leaving.

It seemed that we had finally turned a corner. I hoped my life would start to get back to normal and I could give my actual full-time job at Brigham my full attention again.

On the fourth successful day in a row of treatment, I received an email that was addressed to all of the doctors and nurses on Janel's treatment team. It was from a name I didn't recognize.

> I would like to suggest that we have a team meeting very soon to discuss the treatment and management of patient Janel. We are increasingly challenged in managing him in the infusion room with concerns regarding his safety, our ability to communicate with him, and whether this is a treatment that the patient really wants.

The email signature said the person was an oncology supervisor. What had led to this? The previous emails had suggested that things were going well, and I hadn't heard of any problems from Anne or Hermide. I wrote to the oncology doctors separately from the supervisor who had sent the email. I acknowledged that Janel's care had been challenging, but things seemed to be going better. I wrote that I didn't think the supervisor was in a position to state whether Janel did or didn't want treatment—we had clarified that with him and Wilner long ago. I asked whether they would be willing to be a united front with me in advocating for Janel's care in spite of whatever concerns were being raised.

The oncologist overseeing Janel's care replied that Janel had come alone to chemotherapy the day before. Janel was unable to confirm his name—a safety requirement before receiving chemotherapy—and Hermide wasn't there to speak for him. He then stood up and wouldn't sit back down. The nurses raised the concern that he was there alone, which they didn't think was safe.

How had he ended up there alone? I called Anne. Apparently Thursday was the only day when Hermide wasn't available, so Anne had organized a Creole-speaking volunteer to spend the day with Janel at Brigham after Hermide dropped him off. When the volunteer introduced herself to the interpreter, the interpreter said she wasn't needed and sent her away. It had all been a misunderstanding.

I explained all of this to Janel's oncologist, apologizing that it was the first Thursday that we'd recruited a volunteer and there had been a miscommunication, so I hoped this would go more smoothly in the future.

She replied:

> Thanks, I think that if we ensure that Janel can be accompanied to all visits, they will be fine with treating him.

But there turned out to be larger concerns.

The next morning I met with the supervisor who had written to me. On my way to the meeting, I realized I felt as though I was going to be in the hot seat. My impulse was to passionately defend Janel in the face of potential discrimination against him as a poor foreign patient getting free care, and a difficult patient at that. *Don't do it*, I told myself.

I'd been brash in the face of every concern so far, blinded by my belief that I was acting as a strong advocate for my patient against resistance in the system. But at every step I'd been burned by the practical realities of caring for Janel—most recently, the practical realities that the oncology staff had warned us about before Janel began his treatment. Of course if I hadn't pushed for Janel to get his care in the US, it never would've happened. If I had capitulated to challenges that emerged at each step along the way, I would have been giving up on his life. I had fought hard to do what I believed was the right thing for Janel. But did I really know the right way to do it? The answer was starting to look like a humbling no.

I arrived at the meeting wrestling with these thoughts. Three people were sitting around the table. The supervisor who had sent the email was an older woman in business attire with a yellow legal pad, pen, and her phone set out neatly in front of her. Two of Janel's oncology nurses sat next to her, young women in bright, colorful scrubs. We introduced ourselves, and the supervisor began listing her concerns. Did Janel really want this treatment? Did he really have the mental capacity to consent to it? Did Hermide speak for him and consent for him? If so, how could they get his daily consent for chemotherapy if she wasn't there? And was Hermide really able to manage him at home?

I sat silently, listened, and nodded. These were all valid concerns. And I shared them. She finished, and it was my turn to speak.

"If I can provide some background," I began, not really knowing what I would say next. "Janel comes from one of the poorest parts of Haiti. I don't claim to be able to truly understand him or where he comes from. And I also agree it's a real challenge to not be able to communicate with him directly." I paused. "But believe me, we shared all of these concerns and had local mental health practitioners meet with him in Haiti to assess his capacity and his wishes. Otherwise we wouldn't have brought him here. Our team had extensive discussions with Janel's family and caretakers in Haiti before he came to the US, after he arrived, and again last week when we didn't understand why he was resisting his treatment. They affirmed their understanding of the risks and benefits of treatment, and that Janel would want to do whatever it took to be cured of his disease. They said they wanted Hermide to be as firm with him as she would be with a child since he seems to prefer being curled up in bed rather than engaging with his care." I paused again.

The nurses nodded.

"I know this week didn't go that smoothly, but it went much better than last week, right?" I asked.

"He's done very well with radiation," one of the nurses said. "Sometimes I need to coax him on and off the table, but he lies still and tolerates the mask."

"He needs time to get used to the chemo suite and some encouragement," the other nurse said. "But eventually he participates and allows me to access his port."

The supervisor looked at each nurse and then back at me.

"We saw this week that with encouragement we could do almost a full week of chemotherapy and radiation," I offered.

"We can try to keep going with this," said the supervisor. "But we need someone to be there to consent for chemo if he's not going to talk."

"The only day Hermide can't be there is Thursdays—" I began.

"Then he can't get chemo those days if he's not going to speak," the supervisor said sternly.

I felt my face flush as the fight-or-flight response I'd experienced on my way to the meeting arose. I paused a moment to let it pass. Instead of explaining our plan to have a volunteer with Janel on Thursdays, I said, "Let me check with his oncologist, but I think we can adjust the schedule if needed."

She nodded once and made a note on her legal pad.

"With regard to Hermide," I said, "this has definitely been hard for her, but she is not alone. There are several women who live with her and help her. They're committed to getting Janel through the next few weeks."

"She's very gracious," one of the nurses said, "but this seems like a lot for her."

"Fortunately, she has a lot of experience," I said, trying to allay the concern, though I fully agreed with it.

Silence.

"So can we see how next week goes and then touch base?" I asked.

"I suppose we can try," the supervisor said.

"Thank you," I said and smiled.

The supervisor forced a stale smile back. I could tell she wasn't happy with this, and I couldn't blame her. But she was willing to go along with it, and I was grateful for that.

As everyone started to get up to leave, I couldn't resist giving a little tug on their humanitarian heartstrings. "Just think how amazing it is," I began, "that this young man from one of the poorest places in the world can receive such incredible care at one of the world's best cancer centers. His family in Haiti is very grateful to you, and so are we."

How could anyone argue with that?

The following day, Janel refused to get out of the car again. I was teaching a group of medical students that morning, so my phone was on silent. Afterward, I saw several missed calls from Hermide.

As I walked from the medical school to my clinic, I read an email from one of Janel's nurses, whom Hermide had called when she couldn't reach me. The nurse had come out to the car to try to coax Janel out as I had done several days prior. Janel nodded yes when the nurse asked him if he wanted to come into the hospital, and nodded yes again when she asked if he wanted to get his treatment, but then he wouldn't move. He didn't say anything.

The nurse wrote to us:

> I tried to be verbally firm—no use. I tried to be verbally warm
> and supportive (reminding him of the cookies and drinks
> he enjoys)—no use. This went on for approximately forty
> minutes. We determined any further efforts to try and
> extract him from the car were starting to feel too aggressive.
> We discussed with Hermide that we cannot force Janel
> to participate in care and that she would have to take him
> back home. She was disappointed in the outcome, and left
> with Janel.

I called Hermide.

"No luck today?" I asked.

"No!" she said sharply, at a high pitch, cutting off the word crisply.
It was a way of intoning "no" that I recognized from Haiti when someone was angry, excited, or both. "Do you know what he said to me this
morning?! He said, 'If you think I'm getting up and going, then my
name is not Janel!' Can you believe it? Mm! What are we going to do
now? The nurses said he has the *right to refuse*." She drew out the last
three words as if bracketing them in quotation marks. "I don't want to
hijack him anymore. I *can't* hijack him anymore."

"I'm so sorry," I said, feeling it fall flat. "Did you try calling Wilner?"

"Not today, no. I think we should admit Janel to the hospital. Or
a nursing home. Once he's in the hospital, he's fine. Can we get the
money to do that?"

"I don't know. It would be a last resort," I said. "Can we try one more
time tomorrow? Can we try with Wilner on the phone like last week?"
I felt like I was begging her. I also felt like I shouldn't be begging her. I
had no idea what I would be doing if I were in her shoes. Just hearing
about these challenges over the phone and trying to troubleshoot was
overwhelming me, and that wasn't even one percent of what Hermide
was dealing with.

"We can try," she said, "but I don't think he's going to do it. I've tried everything. And I'm not going to hijack him anymore!" She exhaled a strong sigh. "It just doesn't feel right," she said in a more subdued, sad tone.

"I understand," I replied. "Let's give it one more try. He was doing so well last week, and he really needs this treatment. The tumor is very aggressive."

"We can try," she said, her tone conveying she wasn't optimistic.

"Thank you, Hermide. I'm really sorry this has been so hard. Let me know if I can do anything," I offered, knowing there was nothing I could do.

"I will," she said, knowing the same thing.

I had managed to convince her to persist. But I wasn't sure I was still convinced we were doing the right thing. If Janel could convey that he understood that this treatment was to prolong his life and reduce the risk of his tumor recurring, and if he could articulate that he wanted to stop treatment nevertheless, then we would say he had the capacity to refuse care. We would stop the treatment and fly him home to Haiti. But Janel didn't speak, and we didn't know what he understood. He had said before the surgeries that Wilner could speak for him, and Wilner insisted that Janel would want the treatment. But Janel's behavior was more like a child's most of the time. If a child didn't want to take a medicine, we wouldn't consider the child as having the capacity to refuse. But even if Janel acted like a child, he was a twenty-three-year-old man, and none of us felt comfortable forcing him against his will, even if we believed it was for his own benefit.

The next morning, Hermide called Wilner and left the phone with Janel. When she came back to retrieve the phone, Wilner told her that Janel had agreed to go to treatment. After Hermide hung up, Janel said to Hermide, "I want to go to treatment today."

But then he refused to get out of bed.

Hermide called me.

I was with a patient and silenced my phone so I could call her back when I finished, but she kept calling. I excused myself apologetically and stepped out of the clinic room into the hallway to take the call. I took a deep breath before I answered—the constant disruptions were beginning to wear on me. I was in awe of Hermide's patience and persistence, and I wanted to be helpful, but I didn't really know what I could do—and Janel was not my only patient to take care of.

"I give up," Hermide said and sighed. "We need to get his mother here. Maybe he'll listen to her?"

I told her I would talk with Michelle and Anne to come up with a solution.

Despite our best efforts to get Janel his treatment, it was becoming clear that our strategies to do so were failing. Now what? His mom didn't have a birth certificate, so waiting for a passport and visa for her could take months, as it did for Janel. Should we send him back to Haiti for a few months to recover and then have him come back with his mom when she finally got a passport?

The radiation oncologist thought the sporadic doses of radiation Janel had received over the prior two weeks would contribute to the overall limit he could tolerate before risking toxicity but probably wouldn't contribute much to controlling his tumor if there was a months-long delay before he got further radiation. In other words, if we took a break, the treatment he had received so far would be wasted and couldn't be repeated.

It seemed as though we had to go with our last resort: to hospitalize Janel for the next month so he could receive his full treatment course. Most of the challenges had been at Hermide's, so hopefully everything would go more smoothly if we admitted him to the hospital.

I stepped back into my clinic room, apologized to the patient, and finished the appointment. Despite having fallen way behind, before I called in the next patient, I dashed off emails to Janel's oncology team and to Anne and Michelle about the possibility of admitting Janel to the hospital. Then I kept on seeing patients, and after each one, I checked my email and found a dozen messages flying back and forth discussing what to do next.

"Who will pay if we admit him?" asked one of the oncologists.

"If this is medically necessary for him, then it's part of his care, which the hospital committed to," I replied.

In a separate email chain, Michelle wrote, "I like the idea of admitting him!"

"The hospital administration didn't budget for this—they are not going to be happy with us," I lamented in my reply.

"They can afford it!" she quipped back.

"Agreed, but will they ever want to help us again with another case after this one?" I asked. "This is becoming a disaster!"

We all agreed our only choice was to hospitalize Janel, but this still didn't resolve the question of whether he really wanted to be treated. Anne called Wilner and explained the situation. He again expressed that he was embarrassed about how Janel was behaving and was sure that it was the disease causing him to behave this way. Wilner reiterated that Janel and his family would want us to do everything we could to try to make him disease-free for the future, and he fully supported admitting Janel to the hospital if that was what he needed. Wilner's only concern about hospitalizing Janel was whether the hospital staff would be as patient and kind with Janel as Hermide and the women who lived with her had been. We assured him they would.

Finally, after an exchange of more than forty emails over several hours, we had made a decision and arranged the logistics. Janel would come into the hospital the next day to complete the rest of his six-week course of chemotherapy and radiation therapy.

We were all relieved. A rest for Hermide and the women who helped her take care of Janel. A safer plan to ensure the continuity of Janel's treatment schedule for the oncology staff. A break for Anne, Michelle, and me, from what had been a nearly full-time job of interfacing with Hermide, the oncology staff, and each other to try to make things work in parallel with our full-time jobs in the hospital. And most important, Janel would get the treatment he needed for his tumor in what seemed to be a more comfortable environment for him.

By the time all of this had been sorted out and I had finished seeing all of my patients and writing my clinic notes, it was late in the evening. As I walked home through the cold winter night, I went through my mental checklist for what I needed to pack and take care of before I left for Haiti the next morning for one of my regularly scheduled trips. After weeks of chaos—not to mention the bitter cold of Boston's winter—escaping to Haiti felt like a welcome reprieve.

10

My flight to Haiti was delayed, landing at the same time as flights of several other airlines. The customs hall clearly wasn't prepared for this. I waited in line for almost two hours in the crowded, humid room. If it got much later, I would have to spend the night in Port-au-Prince and travel to Mirebalais the next morning, since navigating the mountain roads at night is dangerous. But so is Port-au-Prince. I was getting anxious.

Finally I made it to the front of the line. I approached the window and gave the customs agent my passport.

"What are you doing in Haiti?" she asked in thickly accented English, thumbing through my passport without looking up.

"Mwen doktè. M travay Zanmi Lasante," I answered. ("I'm a doctor. I work for Partners In Health.")

She continued looking through my passport, not impressed in the least with my credentials or my Creole.

"And what type of doctor?" she asked in English.

"Newolog," I said. ("Neurologist.")

"Ki sa ki yon newolog?" she asked with continued lack of interest. ("And what's a neurologist?") She started entering information into her computer.

I took a moment to think of how to say what I wanted to say in Creole. *"Newolog se doktè pou pwoblem nan tèt,"* I finally said, tapping my finger against my temple and smiling. ("A neurologist is a doctor for problems in the head.")

Now she looked at me, her face suddenly brightening. *"Se doktè tèt ou ye?!"* she asked excitedly, breaking from her previously serious official-border-agent demeanor. ("So you're a head doctor?!")

"Doktè tèt, wi," I replied. ("A head doctor, yes.") I smiled again, amused by the literal translation, "Doctor Head."

She smiled too. *"Eske ou ka we boul m gen nan tèt mwen?"* she asked. ("Could you have a look at this bump in my head?") She leaned forward and pulled apart some strands of hair just before they entered her tight ponytail. She took my index finger and guided it to a small, soft bump on her scalp. *"Kisa m gen la?"* she asked, furrowing her brow in concern. ("What do I have there?") She moved my finger back and forth over the bump. It felt like a pimple or a bug bite, but I wasn't sure.

"Sorry, I'm not the kind of doctor you need. I'm a doctor for what's *inside* the head," I told her.

"M pa gen pwoblem nan tèt mwen?!" she asked, looking surprised and relieved. ("I don't have a problem in my head?!")

"Boul la pa nan tèt, no," I assured her. ("The bump is not inside your head, no.")

"Mesi anpil!" she said. ("Thank you so much!") She stamped my passport with an enthusiastic flourish and handed it back to me with a broad smile.

My first consult of the trip, I joked to myself as I walked past the two-banjo-one-accordion-two-percussion welcome band playing at the entrance to baggage claim.

Once I found the driver and we were on our way, I leaned my head back against the headrest and closed my eyes. The interaction with the customs agent reminded me of a patient I had seen on a previous trip to Haiti who had wanted to be evaluated by a neurologist because she thought her brain was coming out of her nose. It turned out it wasn't her brain, just some mucus—she had sinusitis. We didn't know how or where she had gotten the idea that the mucus coming out of her nose was her brain, but she was very relieved when we told her that her brain was just fine. Maybe the customs agent had similarly thought she had some dangerous growth coming out of her head.

I remembered a conversation I'd had with Dr. Kerling Israel—a leader in Haitian medical education working at PIH/ZL—on one of my first trips to Haiti. Kerling had told me how important she thought neurology training was for Haiti. I presumed she meant because there was only one neurologist in the whole country, leaving patients with limited access to neurologic care and patients' doctors with no training from neurologists. Yes, she acknowledged, doctors in Haiti often failed their patients with neurologic disorders because they had minimal training in how to diagnose and treat these conditions. But she saw the problem as much larger than that.

"Many Haitian patients seek help from traditional healers like voodoo priests," she explained, "especially for neurological problems like seizures and paralysis that can look so strange—like spirit possession—to patients and their families. If a patient comes to our hospital with a neurological problem and the doctor isn't able to provide a diagnosis or treatment, the patient will think, *This is not a problem that can be taken care of by a medical doctor.* So the patient will go to the traditional healers only and may never come back for primary care or prenatal care or surgery or anything. We might even lose these patients from the entire healthcare system. We need to improve our neurologic care in Haiti not just so we can help these patients but so we don't alienate them from the whole medical system by our lack of knowledge in this area. So neurology is a big priority for us."

Neurology in Haiti had seemed to me to be so small and inconsequential compared to huge problems like tuberculosis, AIDS, and malnutrition. But Kerling suggested it was important in ways I hadn't imagined. Her perspective was an inspiring and humbling welcome to my work with her and PIH/ZL in Haiti.

———————

The wards at HUM are housed in a square section of the building with an outdoor courtyard at its center. In the courtyard, a flower garden surrounds a concrete fountain with a small stone footpath leading to it. During my first visits to HUM, the fountain had fish in it, but they had since disappeared. Someone told me they had been stolen.

During my first morning back at HUM, one of the medical residents named Nathalie asked for my help in evaluating an eighteen-year-old patient named Francky. She led me to his bed, which was in the corner of the adult ward, right next to the nurses' station. At first glance, Francky looked like a healthy young man. He was tall enough to fill the hospital bed and appeared fit and strong in a tight white tank top and jeans. He was chatting and laughing with family members, who were sitting on and around his bed. Nathalie asked Francky what had brought him to the hospital.

He said he had developed a headache about a month ago. Over the last week, he had gone blind. His headache had gotten worse too, and his neck had become stiff and painful to move. The resident asked if he'd had any fevers. He said he hadn't.

As I looked at his eyes while he spoke, I noticed he didn't move them at all, and his pupils were fully dilated. When Nathalie shined a light on his pupils, they didn't constrict. She asked him to follow her finger with his eyes.

"I can't see," he reminded her.

She apologized.

"No problem," he said and chuckled gently.

She asked him to look to his left and right, but his eyes didn't move. She asked him to touch his chin to his chest, but he couldn't—his neck was as stiff as a board. Otherwise, he looked well. He had no problem speaking, and he had full strength in his arms and legs.

As Nathalie took out her stethoscope and reflex hammer to examine

Francky, I looked up at the row of patient beds that stretched beyond him. In the next bed, an elderly sunken-eyed man lay sleeping on his side, his tightly distended, pregnant-appearing abdomen starkly off-setting his emaciated chest, which was so thin that every rib was visible. Three flies landed on his belly, flew above it and regrouped, landed again. The man's arm hung limply over the side of his bed, his dangling hand held by a young woman sitting on the floor who was cleaning under each of his fingernails with her own thumbnail.

I looked back at Francky. In contrast to his neighbor, he looked healthy and vibrant. His symptoms had evolved too slowly for a stroke but seemed too quick in progression for a tumor. He hadn't had any fever to suggest an infection, and an HIV test had been negative.

After Nathalie finished examining him, she and I went to look at his CT scan at the nurses' station. I was unsure of what we would find. The first thing that jumped out as Nathalie slowly scrolled down from the top of his brain was that his ventricles—the fluid-filled cavities deep in the brain—were massively enlarged: hydrocephalus, like Janel had. But why? Continuing to scroll through the scan, we discovered the reason. The left half of the cerebellum was massively swollen, so swollen that it was compressing the outflow of the ventricles. In the center of the swelling was a tumor about the size of an olive.

The tumor must have been there much longer than the month during which Francky had developed symptoms. So why had things progressed so rapidly over the last week? The pressure in and around his brain must have reached a tipping point, first causing headaches, then causing compression of all the nerves to his eyes, leading to blindness and his inability to move them. Although the blindness was probably the most concerning to Francky, it was his profound neck stiffness that was most worrisome to me. This signified that the tumor and the pressure it was causing were crowding the foramen magnum. Meaning "great opening" in Latin, the foramen magnum is the passageway through which the spinal cord exits the base of the skull. If the swelling increased any further, vital brain regions that controlled his heart rate and breathing would be crushed as the great opening closed off. This would be fatal.

Since Francky had become blind over the preceding week, it was possible his vision could be restored by removing the tumor. I saw the possibility for a big save here, a much more straightforward one than Janel. Francky's surgery would not be nearly as complex as Janel's had been, and Francky looked so well compared to Janel. But the need for surgery in Francky's case was more urgent than it had been with Janel, since Francky's symptoms had emerged and worsened so rapidly. We had gotten Janel successfully to the US, so hopefully we could pull it off for Francky too.

Nathalie explained to Francky that he had a brain tumor and needed surgery. They told him that I was visiting from Boston and had recently gotten another patient in his situation free surgery in the US, and would try to arrange this for him. I asked Francky if he had a passport. He did. This was great news—the passport had been a rate-limiting step for months in Janel's case. We prescribed steroids to reduce the swelling around the tumor, hoping to alleviate his headache and give us some time to try to find a solution.

It didn't seem like the right moment to ask Brigham to provide free care for another patient from Haiti. Janel had just been admitted for a month of chemotherapy and radiation, and the complexity and cost of his care was far exceeding what any of us had anticipated.

I asked a doctor visiting HUM from another US hospital if she would be willing to contact one of her neurosurgery colleagues back in the States. I sent her some cell phone pictures of the CT scan to pass along. Her neurosurgeon colleague replied to us that the young man absolutely needed surgery and asked if it could be done in Haiti. We said it couldn't and asked if he would consider bringing the patient to his hospital in the US. He didn't reply.

I would be spending the following week teaching at one of the other

PIH/ZL-supported hospitals in a different part of Haiti, but I assured Nathalie I would keep working on trying to get Francky to the US and keep her posted.

While I was at the other site, Nathalie wrote to me that a radiologist from another US hospital was visiting HUM. She asked the radiologist to show the scan to his neurosurgical colleagues back home. The radiologist replied that he couldn't say whether the tumor was operable without an MRI and so he didn't think it was worth showing the CT scan to any surgeons. I disagreed. Although an MRI would certainly help us better define the tumor, even without it, it was clear that this patient needed urgent surgery.

I asked Nathalie to tell the radiologist that a visiting neurologist had seen the patient and his CT scan and was sure the patient needed surgery, so we would appreciate if he could show it to neurosurgical colleagues from his institution to see if they might be able to help. Nathalie went back to the radiologist and tried again, but this time he told her that he thought the tumor was inoperable based on the CT scan. She interpreted this as the radiologist simply not wanting to get involved. Frustrated by the interaction, she gave up on trying to convince him to help us.

I called Anne in Boston to see what she thought we should do. She agreed that it probably was not a good time to ask Brigham about another case when things had not gone as planned with Janel—who, by the way, was doing okay with his treatment in the hospital, she said. But she thought that at eighteen years old, Francky was not necessarily too old to ask for help from a children's hospital she had worked with in the past for surgical cases from Haiti. Anne contacted a neurosurgeon at the hospital, and he agreed that the patient needed urgent surgery. He copied in one of his hospital's administrators to see if free care could be arranged. The administrator sent us a set of forms, and we filled them out and sent them right back. It looked like we had a promising path for Francky, and I called Nathalie to let her know.

She said she would relay the good news to Francky, who fortunately had remained stable over the week I had been at the other site. He was still blind and still had a headache and a stiff neck, but he was still able to eat, talk, and move normally. I was headed back to Boston but promised her I would keep in touch about the plan.

As I sat with my backpack and suitcase waiting for my ride to the airport, two conflicting feelings dueled in my mind: I felt bad that I was going home and I was glad to be going home.

My trips to Haiti always felt so short, and I knew I could do more if I lived and worked there full-time. The one neurologist in Haiti had recently fallen ill, meaning that by leaving I was decreasing the number of practicing neurologists there by 100 percent, from one to zero. Back in Boston I was one among hundreds. It didn't seem right. But I was also eager to return to my Boston life—Nina, my fulfilling new job at Brigham, the basic comforts we take for granted. And this made me feel guilty.

I liked to think that I could adapt well to life in rural Haiti. Although the frequent power outages, blistering heat, oppressive humidity, and lack of air-conditioning and hot water seemed to frustrate some visiting staff, I always enjoyed my time there. But it's easy to adapt to anything for two or three weeks. I am well aware that my colleagues in Haiti have to live with this reality all the time.

Almost every year, one of our Haitian physician colleagues moves to the US. Since they can't work as doctors in the US without repeating all of their training, many go back to school and become nurses. I've heard my US colleagues criticize them. "I thought they were so committed to Haiti. How can they leave? Haiti needs them! What a waste of all their public education!" Easy for us to say, we who come and go, who can be evacuated if something doesn't go according to plan, who can rough it for a few weeks at a time, knowing we're returning to air-conditioning and hot showers, to say nothing of paved roads and continuous electricity. If the opportunity arises for our Haitian colleagues to move to a place with better schools for their children and better healthcare for their families—not to mention safe drinking water from the tap and political stability—how can we fault them?

I heard a car horn beep, and the security guard opened the gate to let the driver in. It was one of HUM's larger vans with two benches along the windows in the back. I pushed my suitcase between the benches, shut the rear doors, and climbed into the passenger seat. Then we waited.

Ten minutes.

Fifteen minutes.

The driver got a few calls, but his Creole was too fast for me to understand what he was saying.

We continued to wait there, engine idling.

Twenty minutes.

Thirty minutes.

I tried to ask if we were waiting for others—maybe that was why he had come in a van instead of a car?—but again, he spoke too quickly for me to understand.

I started to worry that we could be late for my flight. And then I started to worry that since we could be late, the driver would drive quickly and recklessly to avoid being late. I had been in that uncomfortable situation before.

I heard the rear doors of the van open. I looked over my shoulder to see several of the women who work in the staff house piling into the back seat. They left the doors open. A few minutes later, another car pulled up. They loaded some things into the back of the van, but I couldn't see exactly what they were. Then, finally, we left.

Running late, we took the winding, perilous mountain roads at dizzying speeds. When we finally descended onto the straight, flat stretch that leads from the base of the mountains into Port-au-Prince, I was relieved that we'd made it in one piece. The driver floored it, weaving erratically past trucks, *taptaps*, and motorcycles on the crowded street.

A chicken scampered out onto the road ahead. The driver beeped but didn't slow down. The chicken darted back and forth on the road in panicked confusion. At the last moment, it flapped its wings into clumsy flight, bounced off the grill of a truck coming in the opposite direction with a hard smacking sound, got thrown to the ground, and was run over by our van with a loud thud.

As I winced at the sound of our tire crushing the chicken, the women in the back of the van burst out laughing.

"*O O! Li mouri!!*" one exclaimed, trying to catch her breath from laughing so hard. ("Oh-oh! It died!")

"*Li mouri?*" another asked, laughing. ("Did it die?")

"*O wi, li mouri!*" the first woman said emphatically. ("Oh yes, it died!")

This made the other woman laugh even more. "*O Ooooo! Li mouriiiiii!!*"

They took turns explaining what happened. "We ran it over!" one said. "No," another said, "it flew into the other car and died!" "No," the third woman said, "it bounced off the truck and then we ran it over and that killed it."

They argued playfully about it, their laughter punctuated by school-girlish squeals of "*O O!*" and "*Li mouri!*"

I felt slightly nauseated. I wasn't sure if it was the thump I'd heard and felt as we ran over the poor bird or if I was just getting carsick from the vertiginous speed at which we'd just spun through the mountain roads and our start-and-stop weaving in and out of city traffic. I gritted my teeth and squeezed my eyes shut against the queasiness, hoping we'd be at the airport soon.

The ladies were still giggling away. It felt odd to keep hearing the phrase "It died!" accompanying such joyful laughter, not that I would have expected a somber period of mourning for a road kill.

I thought of how one of my American colleagues in Haiti described what happens when a patient dies in the hospital here, a sadly common occurrence due to how sick patients often are by the time they make it to the hospital and the limitations of locally available treatments when they finally do arrive.

"It's always the same scene," my colleague had said with jaded authority. "The patient is pronounced dead. The family wails dramatically in the courtyard for a few minutes. Then they compose themselves, come in, cover the body with a white sheet, take it outside, put it in the back of their car, and drive home to plan the funeral. It's like they're just used to death here because they see it so much."

Used to death? It's true that death occurs more commonly at all ages in Haiti compared to the US. Infants born in Haiti are eight times more likely to die than infants born in the US. Pregnant women in Haiti are twenty-five times more likely to die than pregnant women in the US. And the average life expectancy in Haiti is just sixty-four years—fourteen years less than on the same island across the border in the Dominican Republic and sixteen years less than in the US. But I thought it was insensitive and ignorant to imply that Haitians could get used to watching their loved ones die, their children and mothers and fathers and friends taken from them too soon.

My colleague's comments reminded me of how after the 2010 earthquake killed hundreds of thousands and left more than a million homeless, nearly every article described the "resilience of the Haitian people." A compliment at first glance, and one with some truth to it—Haitians and Haiti have survived countless disasters, both natural and unnatural. But as one journalist noted, "Sometimes compassion can be a form of contempt." In a cynical piece on post-earthquake reporting entitled "How to Write About Haiti," another journalist mocked the resilience trope as follows:

You are struck by the 'resilience' of the Haitian people. They will survive no matter how poor they are. They are stoic, they rarely

*complain, and so they are admirable. The best poor person is one
who suffers quietly. A two-sentence quote about their misery fitting
neatly into your story is all that's needed.*

How could we outsiders know what's happening beneath the surface
of so-called stoic, silent suffering in a culture that is not our own?

I wondered if my colleague would interpret the ladies' laughter at
the chicken's death as symbolic of Haitians taking death more lightly
since they are "used to" it. But there is always a risk of misinterpreting
something that may have a completely different meaning—or perhaps
no meaning at all—in another culture.

When we arrived at the airport, I thanked the driver and went
around to the back of the van to get my luggage. One of the ladies sitting in the back opened the rear doors from the inside and slid my
suitcase out to me. I thanked her and reached in to grab it. On the floor
next to the suitcase were two large chickens tied together at the legs and
wings. I couldn't tell if they were dead or alive. Next to them was a large
bucket of raw meat on ice.

The women saw me looking at the chickens and meat, and laughed.
"*Se pa pou w,*" one teased. ("That's not for you.") They knew I was vegan,
and they kindly made non-meat, non-dairy portions for me at each
meal when I was working at HUM. They told me they were cooking for
an event in Port-au-Prince later that day. I smiled, thanked them, and
headed into the airport terminal.

———————

After landing in Boston, I received this email from Nathalie:

Hi Aaron,

Our patient is in pain, we had to put more morphine in his
treatment.

He is still conscious but sleeps more and more.

The family is putting on a lot of pressure. We are telling them
that there is still hope . . . It's hard for them though. But I
know it takes time . . .

Nathalie

The fact that Francky was sleeping more and more suggested the
pressure inside his skull was worsening, causing compression of the
consciousness centers of his brain.

We were running out of time.

Anne and I wrote to the administrative contact at the hospital that
had offered to help us with Francky's case. We explained that the patient was getting worse and asked whether there was any progress on
the possibility of free care. The reply:

I am not aware about free care. This can be discussed with my
manager.

Clearly there had been a miscommunication. Why had we filled
out all of that paperwork if not for a free-care request? The emails had
seemed pretty clear from our perspective. There must have been some
sort of misunderstanding.

Anne wrote back, asking how to contact the administrator's manager.
The next morning, I awoke to find this email:

Hi Aaron,

I'm sorry I have very bad news.

Our patient Francky just died from respiratory failure.

He was really in pain so I guess it's better for him . . .

Take care,

Nathalie

I was devastated. He was only eighteen. Eighteen! In so many other places in the world he'd have had surgery before it was too late. He'd have had the chance to become an adult. Instead, *li mouri*—he died. Like the chicken on the road to Port-au-Prince, Francky was in the wrong place at the wrong time. And so—*"O O! Li mouri"*—he died. He died what Paul Farmer, one of PIH's founders and leaders, calls a "stupid death"—a tragically unnecessary death in a poor country from a condition that would have never been fatal in a rich country.

I was quick to blame the administrative delays for Francky's stupid death. But Anne felt that was unfair. "We only had a month from the time you met him to his death," she said, "and that is faster than any diagnosis-to-surgery time that I've ever had with these cases, other than post-earthquake. Even if they had accepted him right away, we would have needed a team to get a visa for him and make all the arrangements that you know took forever with Janel."

Anne was right. It wasn't "the system"—which it was my knee-jerk response to rage against—but "The System": the lack of some type of global effort to address the inequities in access to medical care that cause treatable patients like Francky to die stupid deaths, and patients like Janel to wait so long for care that it could be too late to help them in any meaningful way.

I wrote to Nathalie, feeling my attempt at an apology fall flat:

> That is devastating news to hear. I am so sorry and so sad
> that we could not make this happen. I and another colleague
> kept pushing the administration at the hospital that was
> considering it, but unfortunately I/we/they could not move
> it along. We will gently let them know the consequences of
> their delays and hopefully be better equipped to act quickly
> next time. I am so sorry that we could not come through
> for the patient . . . I assure you it wasn't from lack of trying,
> but it feels empty for all of us to say that. The machine is a
> very slow-moving one here—it took us three months to get

another patient here. I feel bad that he died with him and his family having a sense of hope that we could have done more. We surely hoped so too, and I am sorry we failed him and them.

She replied:

Don't worry. We all know that you did everything you could and I really thank you for that. And administration had also to do its work. I think there is nothing that could have prevented this sad ending.

As you said, I have the same feeling of guilt because of the hope we gave to the family. I didn't dare talk with the mom, I felt so bad . . .

C'est la vie . . .

I hope next time it will work out.

We'll do better, I believe in us ;)

Thank you one thousand times for your support. See you soon.

11

For the first few days after Janel was readmitted to the hospital, he mostly slept. During the rare moments when he was awake, he didn't speak and barely moved. He just stared straight ahead, blinking rarely. Daily brain radiation and chemotherapy are exhausting for patients, but Janel's state was far beyond what would be expected for treatment side effects. Still, the fact that he could consistently receive his medical care every day without incident meant that we were achieving our goal: to give him the best chance at the longest possible recurrence-free survival.

While I was still in Haiti trying to find a solution for Francky, Michelle had sent me a text message with a cell phone video attached. In the frozen first frame, Janel is standing in a hallway at Brigham between his nurse and physical therapist, each holding one of his arms. He's wearing a white long-sleeved shirt and light blue scrub pants. As the video plays, Janel walks slowly but steadily, the nurse and physical therapist just barely supporting him for balance.

"Janel, salye Doktè Martineau!" Michelle says from near the phone. ("Janel, say hi to Dr. Martineau!") *"Bonjou, Doktè Martineau,"* she half sings, half says to him. ("Hi, Dr. Martineau.")

Slowly, Janel raises his hand and waves. *"Kouman ou ye?"* he hoarsely ekes out. ("How are you?")

"Anfòm," Michelle replies and laughs. ("Fine.")

"Tout bagay byen pou ou?" Janel asks. ("Everything going well with you?")

"Wi!" Michelle replies enthusiastically. ("Yes!")

Janel's face brightens into a broad, full-toothed Cheshire-cat smile. Then he laughs and looks down sheepishly to his left. The video stops with him frozen like that, smiling and looking away bashfully.

I was amazed at how well Janel was doing and watched the video again and again on my phone. I showed it to Martineau.

"Wow," he said, shaking his head in disbelief. "I can't believe how much better he looks!"

"Me neither," I said. I really couldn't believe that he could look so great in the hospital after doing so poorly in the weeks leading up to his admission.

I was eager to see Janel's progress when I returned to Boston, hoping it would help me feel better after Francky's devastating death. But it turned out that Michelle's video had captured a rare good moment.

Janel had fluctuated between extremes over the first weeks of his rehospitalization. There were days when his nurses said he sang and danced with them, winking and making kissy faces. But on most days he simply lay in bed gazing vacantly for the entire day, wide-eyed and unresponsive. Even when he responded with minimal nods of his head, he was not able to clearly indicate whether he knew he was in the hospital or even in the US.

This was how he looked when I went to see him after I got home— exactly the same as before I'd left. I looked through his chart to see what had happened while I was away.

Janel had undergone a follow-up MRI scan that showed no reason for why he was so impaired. The tumor remnant was minuscule, his brain had returned to its normal shape and showed no complications from the surgery, and his ventricles were still normal in size, showing that his shunt was working.

His inpatient oncology team had wondered if he was having non-convulsive seizures—seizures that result in an altered mental state without causing the bodily shaking of typical seizures. But several days of EEG recordings of Janel's brain waves didn't show any signs of seizure activity. The oncologists consulted the psychiatry team.

The psychiatry team thought Janel might be suffering from catatonia, a state categorized by mutism (not speaking), immobility, lack of interaction with the environment, and waxy flexibility (sustaining whatever posture—usually of the limbs—that someone else places the patient in). Catatonia can be seen in psychiatric conditions like schizophrenia, depression, and bipolar disorder, but it can also be caused by neurologic or medical diseases and medications. The psychiatrists tried treating Janel with lorazepam (Ativan). Why a sedative medication should work to resolve a sedated state is unclear, yet it does—improvement with lorazepam actually helps confirm the diagnosis of catatonia. But lorazepam had no effect on Janel. The psychiatry team suggested a neurology evaluation.

Since I was away in Haiti, another neurologist was consulted to evaluate Janel. The neurologist labeled Janel's state as akinetic mutism (literally "non-moving not speaking")—a condition that shares features with catatonia but doesn't include the symptom of waxy flexibility, doesn't respond to lorazepam, and is usually associated with an underlying neurologic disease. The neurologist tried treating Janel with a dopamine-based treatment normally used in patients with Parkinson's disease to see if that would perk him up. This didn't work either.

In cases like Janel's, the artificial boundaries between neurology (the science of the brain) and psychiatry (the science of the mind) are exposed. Was Janel's behavior due to a depressed level of brain function, or was he simply depressed? Was he depressed by his condition, or was he depressed because of his condition? Were his fluctuations a neurologic phenomenon related to his brain's recovery from the tumor and his three surgeries, or a psychological manifestation of being alone, far from home, and confused due to his neurologic impairment? The oncology team and Hermide had taken the approach of treating Janel as if he were behaving like a child. How would a child respond to spending months away from his home and family?

Maybe Janel was simply more susceptible to the fatiguing effects of chemotherapy and brain radiation because his level of neurologic function was diminished from the many years he had lived with the tumor and because he had undergone such extensive brain surgeries. But this wouldn't explain the sporadic good days when he could walk and talk, not to mention sing and dance.

From the beginning, I had known that Janel's surgery could result in one of three outcomes: it could make him better, it could prevent progression of his tumor but without improving his level of function, or, in the worst case, it could make him even worse. On some days, he was definitely much better than before surgery, on some days he was the same, and on some days he seemed worse. But better and worse than what? I realized we never did have a clear understanding of his baseline before he developed the tumor. We had been told that he was normal until about a year before we met him, but the tumor could not have grown so large that fast. And it certainly wasn't normal that he was only in fourth grade at age twenty-three, though that could just as well have been an effect of his poverty rather than his intellectual development.

I wrote to Martineau in Haiti to see if he had any insights into why Janel might be acting the way he was. He didn't, but he was determined to try to figure it out. He set off to retrace Janel's path from the time before he first met him. We hoped that if we could better understand Janel's past, maybe we could begin to make sense of his present.

First, Martineau went to visit Wilner. Wilner had met Janel just over two years before we did, when Janel became involved in his church and decided to convert to evangelism. Over subsequent months, Janel began complaining of headaches that progressively worsened. He went to a local clinic, where a CT scan was recommended, but his family couldn't afford it. Sometime in the next year, Wilner noticed that Janel was no longer coming to church, and he went to look for him. He found

Janel living with his mother and no longer able to take care of himself. He couldn't bathe, dress, or eat on his own, his headaches had become more severe, he had developed trouble walking, and he had begun urinating on himself. Wilner didn't think Janel's mother was able to adequately take care of him due to her living conditions, so he took Janel into his own four-room home, where he lived with his wife and two children. Janel's mother visited him at Wilner's house and helped take care of him. When HUM opened, Wilner took Janel there to be evaluated, and he was finally able to get a CT scan for free. The scan revealed the tumor, and Janel was referred to Martineau.

Wilner didn't know much about Janel's life before he met him, but he gave Martineau directions to Janel's school. It turned out that Janel had gone to school in the region where Martineau had worked for another PIH/ZL hospital for four years before being asked to join the first group of physicians at HUM. Since Martineau was well known in the community, the staff at the school let him look through the archives of report cards to find out which class Janel had last been in. Martineau found the teacher's name, and the staff at the school gave him directions to find the teacher's house.

The teacher explained that Janel lived in a very remote impoverished area with no roads leading to or from it. Janel had to walk several hours to school, traversing a river along the way. When he arrived at school, the teacher thought he seemed "*dans les vapeurs*" ("in the mists"), sometimes staring off. He was slower to learn than the other students. The teacher had presumed all of this was because Janel was tired from walking such a long distance every day, and because he probably went hungry on many days.

Leaving the school, Martineau continued to trace Janel's life path, finding his way to Janel's mother's house. The route took him off the dirt road into a wooded area and over a small stream. When he arrived in Janel's community, Martineau asked an elderly woman to show him which house belonged to Janel's mother. The woman led him to a one-room shack made of crumbling wood panels built on a cracked slab of concrete. The house was empty except for a small mattress on the concrete floor and clothes hanging from the wooden rafters.

Martineau waited for Janel's mother. She arrived with a small black plastic bag of items she'd bought at the market. They spoke in front of her house.

She told Martineau that Janel had been born normally at home. He'd had a normal infancy and childhood, walking and talking at the same age as other children in the community. She described Janel as a sweet child who didn't misbehave. He didn't begin going to school until age twelve. She didn't give a clear reason for this, but Martineau presumed it was because she couldn't afford the school fees, uniforms, and school supplies. Janel had to repeat several years in school multiple times before being allowed to move forward. When his illness began at around age twenty-one, he had reached fourth grade. He failed the exam needed to pass to fifth grade.

From what Martineau was able to piece together, it was possible that Janel's tumor had been there for many years before causing the headaches that led him to seek medical attention. It may have even been the cause of his difficulties in school. But the odd behaviors and drastic fluctuations Janel was exhibiting in Boston were completely new. Were they due to the neurological stresses of the tumor and surgeries, the psychological stresses of being separated from his home and family, or a combination of the two? I didn't know. I just hoped he would improve.

It was May, and Janel was nearing the end of his six weeks of chemotherapy and radiation. As planning began for his discharge from Brigham back to Hermide's until the next round of treatment, I received this email from his oncologist:

> The plan had been to restart chemotherapy about 6 weeks after radiation and do 6 more monthly cycles. It would be

intensive chemotherapy again, typically given outpatient. We
don't know if adjuvant chemotherapy is even needed given
how rare PPTID is. We might be over-treating? On the other
hand, it could increase his chance for cure. There is no data to
guide us unfortunately. Given the difficulties we have faced
until recently and the fact that we are not sure what is the
correct treatment for PPTID, I am inclined to skip this phase
of chemotherapy.

We wanted to give Janel the fullest chance of a cure from his tumor.
His oncologist seemed to be indicating that it wasn't clear how helpful six more months of chemotherapy would be toward that goal since
his tumor was so rare. Did the unclear benefits justify the clear risks?
Beyond the medical considerations, how would he handle another six
months away from home? And would Hermide be willing to take care
of him for six more months?

Despite the waxing and waning of Janel's mental state in the hospital, he hadn't demonstrated any of the challenging behavior he had
at Hermide's. But he also hadn't done so at the rehab facility before he
first went to Hermide's, so we really had no idea what to expect when he
returned to her home. How could we balance the possible, but uncertain, medical benefits of additional chemotherapy with the potential
psychosocial harm of putting him—and Hermide—through what they
had been through before? Six months would be a long time, longer than
the entire period Janel had been in the US up to that point.

I pondered these questions as I sat in a chair next to Janel's hospital
bed at Brigham. Visiting him for a half hour or so each day had become
a ritual I hoped might help to break up the monotony of his life in the
hospital. But I acknowledged it was maybe just as much for me to feel
like I was doing something for him. Having just read the oncologist's
email before visiting him, I wondered if I had spent more time writing
emails and having phone calls and thinking about Janel than I had
actually spent with him.

I looked over at him. He was staring blankly at the muted television, where a daytime talk show's guest laughed silently. He had shaken my hand when I came in, but I hadn't been able to get him to talk to me.

There had been a few fleeting moments over the past months when his toothy grin had shown us that he was in there somewhere. But who was the he in there? Who was this twenty-three-year-old man? Was he scared or sad or homesick? What was he thinking about and dreaming about during these months in the hospital? Could he remember what it was like when he was healthy? What had he talked about and thought about and laughed about then? How would he remember his time in the hospital, in Boston, at Hermide's? Would he remember it at all?

Looking at him, wondering about his inner life, I thought of the Haitian proverb *Tout moun se moun* (Every person is a person). It's a simple phrase, but a radical notion. If every person truly believed that every other person was a person just like them, then how could anybody accept inequity, let alone racism, sexism, classism, and the conflicts that arise as a result of these individual views and societal forces?

Martineau, Hermide, Michelle, Anne, and I were committed to getting Janel the care he needed in spite of all of the obstacles we faced because we held true to this notion. Janel is a person. We were not under any illusion that we could solve the world's inequities, but helping Janel gave us the chance to try to right one individual wrong, to try to rectify one grave inequity. This is the work of PIH that had inspired me to want to work with them: to create systems that help the poorest individuals, to counter the notion that some lives are worth less than others, which Paul Farmer has called "the root of all that's wrong with the world."

Why should the country where Janel was born or his poverty mean he shouldn't receive the highest standard of medical care? On the contrary, PIH defines its mission as providing a preferential option for the poor, since the poor are preferentially affected by disease.

Tout moun se moun. Every person is a person. Somehow the debate about risks and benefits of more chemotherapy seemed less theoretical with this proverb in mind. I couldn't speak Creole well enough to ask Janel what he wanted. He wouldn't have been able to respond anyway. But I thought of how Wilner insisted that Janel and his family wanted to do everything possible in pursuit of a cure, and we had the opportunity to offer that to him.

How were we to know where his fluctuations would land? Maybe there would be more and more good moments as time went on. Or maybe this was how he would spend his years, mostly detached from the world around him but with occasional moments full of life. Either way, didn't he still deserve every chance at a full cure? Who were we to decide if it was too difficult—for him, for Hermide, for the hospital—to continue his treatment? Even if it might be overtreatment, wasn't that better than risking undertreatment? If we could possibly extend his life, why shouldn't we try? A few more difficult months would be a small price to pay for this.

Tout moun se moun. Every person is a person. Yes, that was the principle on which this whole endeavor rested. I decided we shouldn't give up.

I felt moved by my reflections but had no way of sharing them with Janel, no way of asking him what he thought.

"*Dako, Janel, m prale,*" I said, patting him on the hand. ("Okay, Janel, I'm going.")

He didn't react. If he was in there somewhere, I hoped he knew that I would keep fighting for him.

As I exited his hospital room and began washing my hands at a sink in the hallway, I saw one of the oncology professors I had worked with during my internship—the first year of my residency. My internship was the most challenging year of my life. I often spent eighty or more hours per week in the hospital, working thirty-hour shifts, not seeing the light of day for weeks at a time in the depths of the Boston winter. During some of the darkest hours, this oncology professor had been a beacon of warmth and compassion to her interns and to her patients. Her extraordinary bedside manner had reminded me why I was going through the struggles and sleepless nights of this grueling training: to reach her level of skill and grace as a physician.

"What brings you back to the oncology ward?" she asked, smiling softly, cocking her head slightly to the side.

"How much time do you have?" I joked, trying to smile but still very much wrapped up in the reflections that had just moved me at Janel's bedside. "The short story is that we brought a patient here from Haiti for the largest brain tumor any of us had ever seen. It's a pineal tumor so rare most of us had never even heard of it: PPTID—the tumor between pineocytoma and pineoblastoma. Anyway, it took two huge surgeries to get it all out, and then he needed a shunt. Now he's just finishing six weeks of chemo and radiation . . ." I trailed off.

Suddenly I felt shocked and saddened by my words. Had I really processed all that Janel had been through? Running through it out loud gave me pause. I had just decided in my mind that I should fight for him, but did he even want to be a passive recipient of that fight? I realized I didn't know.

I tried to continue. "There are a lot of longer stories in there, but . . ." I broke off again. I was a little choked up. I felt like I had just had some sort of clarity while sitting next to Janel, but now I wondered whether it was really about him or more about me applying the principles to which I aspired in his care. Sure, every person is a person. But does every person need to suffer through an unproven, aggressive chemotherapy regimen more than one thousand miles from home?

My oncologist colleague kept smiling warmly at me, nodding slowly, waiting patiently for me to continue.

I tried again. "He's had . . . a rough course . . . but, well . . . he's . . . I guess he's getting a little better. I mean, he fluctuates, but . . ." I looked up and forced a sad smile. "Anyway, sorry, I'm rambling on. It's kind of a long story."

"Sounds like a journey for him and for you," she said. "You know, I have an oncology colleague who used to work for PIH. I remember how she used to bring chemo over to Rwanda in her suitcase for PIH to treat cancer patients there. It's amazing work you guys do."

I asked her how she was and how her work was going, and tried to listen as she told me. But my thoughts had latched on to what she had just said. Could we give Janel the rest of his chemo in Haiti? He could be with his mother. He could get rehab at HUM. He would surely be much happier at home. Lost in these thoughts, I said goodbye to my former oncology professor and wandered back to my office.

Getting the medications to Haiti and administering them would be no problem. The risk would be if Janel suffered complications from the aggressive chemotherapy. He could be hospitalized at HUM if that happened, but would he have the same chance for a good recovery as in the US? What if they couldn't get the right lab tests or medications? After all he'd been through in the US and all we'd done for him, I didn't want him to die a stupid death from a complication in Haiti that could have easily been managed or prevented in Boston.

I discussed all of this with Anne, Michelle, and Janel's oncologist. Our consensus was that we would let him recover and get rehabilitation in Haiti for the next six weeks, then bring him back to Boston for his first round of chemotherapy to see how he did. If it went well, we could do the rest in Haiti. If there were medical complications, we would have to think about doing the entire six-month course in Boston.

Janel was discharged back to Hermide's house with the plan to get him home the next time PIH had a nurse or doctor traveling from Boston to Haiti who could fly with him. The rehab team at HUM arranged for a bed on the rehab ward to be available for him when he arrived.

Janel mostly slept at Hermide's while awaiting his return to Haiti. There were no struggles.

On the morning of Janel's flight, Anne went to the airport to meet Hermide, Janel, and the doctor who had agreed to have Janel travel with him to Haiti. The doctor was a young man, short-haired, clean-shaven, spectacled, and relaxed. Anne briefed him on Janel's condition and explained that he might have had some seizures after one of his surgeries, but it wasn't certain, and Janel was on an anti-seizure medication just in case.

While Anne spoke, the doctor looked past her at Janel sitting in an airport wheelchair with his usual wide-eyed stare, tufts of hair growing around the large scar across his scalp. Anne thought the doctor looked increasingly uneasy about what he had agreed to. But if he was nervous, he didn't say so. Anne told him not to worry, Janel would probably just sleep for the entire flight. She assured him he could call us if there were any issues.

Two hours later, we received a text message from the young physician:

> The airline crew is a little nervous . . . Any medical information
> I need to be aware of other than what you've passed on?

I couldn't help but wonder who was more nervous, the airline crew or the doctor traveling with Janel. I certainly would have been nervous if I had been asked to travel with a patient I didn't know and couldn't communicate with, especially one who was so neurologically impaired and could have a seizure on the plane. In fact, I would have been nervous to travel with Janel, and I had probably spent more time with him than with any patient I'd ever taken care of. While I was thinking about this, Michelle replied, conveying her usual confidence and optimism that everything would work out just fine:

> They are often nervous ;) Just flash your doctor badge and
> I think they will calm down. His cognitive issues may be what's
> making them worry, but he really should be fine. He was
> admitted for 6 weeks and the only real event was a possible
> seizure, but he is on medication for that, so it should not be
> a problem!

A few minutes later, he replied:

> OK, thanks! I think they're OK: after speaking with six
> different crew members, they are OK, and in any case, the
> airplane is now pushing back from the gate, so we're good.

To everyone's relief, Janel slept through the entire flight and was transported uneventfully to the rehab ward at HUM. Just over five months after Janel had left Haiti for the first time in his life, he was finally home.

Our first report from the rehab team at HUM was that Janel preferred lying in bed and sleeping all day, engaging only intermittently in physical therapy. But the rehab team was persistent, Janel slowly acclimated to the ward, and Janel's mother came to HUM and stayed with him, encouraging him to participate more with his physical therapists. After a few weeks, the rehab team reported to us that he was able to walk the length of the ward and back with minimal support. He was eating on his own and indicating with gestures to the rehab staff when he needed help to get to the bathroom instead of just wetting the bed as he had done when he first arrived.

By the end of six weeks of rehab, Martineau wrote to me how impressed he was with Janel's progress:

> Janel walked over 300 feet with hardly any assistance. He
> can eat on his own with only a small residual tremor. He spoke
> to me in full sentences. I think we've made great strides. We
> must continue to accompany him.

It was starting to look like Janel might turn out to be a big save after all. I was glad we had pushed to get him maximal treatment rather than giving up prematurely.

We had hoped Janel's mother would be able to return to Boston with him, but due to ongoing political chaos in Haiti, Martineau no longer had a personal contact in the immigration office. Despite his best efforts, he was still a long way away from getting her a passport through the normal process. It could take months. Janel would have to return to Boston alone.

Unfortunately, there weren't any PIH staff members traveling between Haiti and Boston around this time to accompany him. I was going back to Haiti the following week to continue my work with Martineau and the HUM medical residents, and so I offered to have Janel fly back with me at the end of my trip. But this would have been too late to make the appointments already scheduled for him at Brigham to resume his treatment. I was disappointed I wouldn't get the chance to see him doing so well in Haiti, but I also felt guiltily relieved that I wouldn't have the somewhat frightening responsibility of flying back with him.

Anne suggested we thank Hermide by paying for a trip to Haiti for her to visit family and friends, then fly back to Boston with Janel. Hermide was happy to do this, and we booked her trip for the following weekend. As it turned out, I left for Haiti on the very same day they were returning to Boston. Looking down on the clouds from 30,000 feet, I thought about the odd coincidence: I was flying from my home in Boston to work in rural Haiti while Janel was flying from his home in rural Haiti to my workplace in Boston, both of us flying to *lòt bò a*— the other side.

12

Late June in Haiti is sweltering. Although June falls during the rainy season, it only rains for about an hour or two each evening. The temperature peaks in the high 90s by midday, the air becoming progressively more humid and heavy until it explodes into a brief but torrential evening downpour. The storm cools things off a bit outside, but the concrete staff house seems to retain the heat from the day. The rains just make it more humid.

As I walked to the hospital in the early morning, my shoes got sucked into the thick, sticky mud from the previous night's rains. Jerking them out made a loud kissing noise, my feet sometimes slipping out of my shoes. I remembered from my visit during the prior year's rainy season that by noon, when I walked back to the staff house for a quick lunch of rice and beans, the dirt road would be dusty and chalky, baked from just a few hours of summer Caribbean sun. Then the nightly rains would turn the route into sludge again, and the process would repeat. *Haiti, land of extremes*, I thought.

My morning ritual in Haiti has always been to get to the hospital about an hour before beginning my work there so I can catch up on the previous day's emails, since the staff house doesn't have internet. I had come to appreciate the internet-free period from sunset to sunrise, which allowed me to either focus more fully on whatever work I had brought with me or get lost in a novel until I sweated myself to sleep under my mosquito net. But I tried to keep up with my Boston life as much as I could while I was in Haiti by responding to emails from 7 to

8 a.m., during the lunch hour, and then at the end of the day before going back to the staff house.

When I arrived at HUM, it was still early, and the cleaning staff was sweeping the hospital floors, humming hymns as they worked. They looked at me as I approached and then down at my mud-caked feet. I scraped the soles of my shoes against the concrete walkway to the entrance to remove some of the mud and then wiped them off on a patch of damp grass.

I made my way up the stairs to the administrative area, found an empty office, flipped on the ceiling fan, sat down, and waited for my phone to connect to the hospital Wi-Fi. I always felt my pulse quicken as I connected to the internet each morning in Haiti, wondering what I might have missed in the last twelve hours at work, at home, in the news. Fortunately, there was usually nothing major.

This morning, as my inbox convulsed with each spurt of new emails, I saw a message from Anne fly by with the subject "Janel" and scrolled down against the incoming tide to open it. The email had been sent just before midnight:

> Hermide and Janel were on the way home from the airport and are now headed to Brigham after Janel had a seizure. Hermide called me soon after they left the airport with concern that he was having some shaking, but it resolved while we were on the phone and we agreed she should continue home. She called again just now to say that he had a big seizure, describing tonic/clonic movements of his arms and legs lasting 2 minutes. Sorry for the news.

Thank goodness this hadn't happened in the air, I thought as I toggled to my phone app for the Brigham medical record system. I imagined the plane making an emergency landing in some small rural airport and taking Janel to the nearest local emergency room. What would they have made of such a complicated patient? I could see the staff's eyes widening as Hermide explained that he'd had several neurosurgeries, radiation, and chemotherapy for a rare brain tumor, that he had a shunt, and that they were flying back from Haiti to Boston for more treatment. And if he had a seizure on an airplane, would everyone have insisted on another air ambulance flight to get him back to Boston—and where would we have come up with another $33,000 to support that? Maybe we would have had to drive down to pick up Janel and Hermide and drive them back. It was concerning that he'd had a seizure, but at least it had happened after the plane had landed in Boston.

I searched for Janel's name in the medical record app. As the slow internet connection loaded his chart, I noticed the location in the hospital listed for him. It wasn't the emergency room—it was the operating room. The pit of my stomach tightened as I read the notes in Janel's chart. He'd had another seizure shortly after arriving in the emergency room and had immediately undergone a CT scan. The scan showed that his ventricles were massively enlarged again. His shunt had malfunctioned. Ian had taken him for emergency surgery to repair or replace it.

Not only were we lucky that this hadn't happened on the plane, we were very lucky this hadn't happened in Haiti. Janel could have died.

I wrote to Ian to see what he thought had happened. Could it have been an effect of the altitude as I had feared could occur on Janel's initial flight from Haiti to Boston months earlier?

"Every once in a while the shunt valves go down," he replied. "It is actually a good opportunity to remove it and do an ETV."

ETV stands for endoscopic third ventriculostomy, an operation in which the neurosurgeon makes a small hole in the skull and passes a metal scope slightly larger than a drinking straw through it into the ventricles of the brain. The scope's tiny camera relays images to a video monitor. The surgeon guides tools through the device to puncture a hole in the floor of one of the ventricles, allowing a new channel for egress of excess fluid. In some cases of hydrocephalus, this detour makes a shunt unnecessary. Because of Janel's shunt failure and the

fear of another shunt complication when he was back in Haiti, we
hoped an ETV would spare him the need for a shunt.

The shunt removal and ETV procedure would be Janel's fourth neurosurgical intervention.

———————

It was my third trip of the year to Haiti to work with Martineau and
the internal medicine residents. The strategy of working regularly and
intensively with a small group of local doctors was paying off. They
could now easily diagnose recurrent one-sided pulsating headaches
accompanied by nausea, photophobia (aversion to bright light), and
phonophobia (aversion to noise) as classic migraines. They knew the
instant they saw the combination of a masklike face, stooped posture,
slow gait, and resting tremor that the patient likely had Parkinson's
disease. They recognized the common story of patients falling unconscious with rhythmic, uncontrolled shaking followed by confusion as
epileptic seizures. And they learned how to treat these conditions with
locally available medications.

Under their care, patients' migraines decreased in severity and
frequency when they were prescribed low-dose amitriptyline and encouraged to stop their near-daily use of aspirin and Tylenol. Patients
who had been stiff, slow, and statue-like from untreated Parkinson's
disease began to move more fluidly and smile more animatedly when
they were prescribed carbidopa-levodopa. Children with epilepsy not
only finally had their seizures controlled with locally available anti-
epileptic medications, like carbamazepine or phenytoin, but were able
to go back to school—local teachers in rural Haiti thought epilepsy
was contagious and often refused to let children with seizures attend.
Patients expressed enormous gratitude, but this was bittersweet—I was
so happy to see them feeling better and returning to their normal lives,
but I found it troubling to think about how long they had suffered from
such easily treatable conditions.

Unfortunately, not all of the patients we saw had such simple solutions.

A thirty-two-year-old single mother named Nadège had been diagnosed with migraines, but her headaches continued to worsen. She had also noticed bulging of her right eye—the medical term is proptosis, which always sounded to me exactly how it appears. She was otherwise perfectly healthy and even still had normal vision in the proptotic eye. Her CT scan revealed a marble-size tumor just behind her eye, pushing it outward and compressing her optic nerve, the conduit of vision from the eye to the brain. Without surgery, the growing tumor would cause the eye to bulge out farther, and she could go blind.

A fifty-three-year-old woman named Jesula also had debilitating headaches. Her CT scan showed a huge meningioma—a tumor of the brain's lining—just below the top of her skull. The tumor had grown so large that all of the fluid-filled spaces in and around her brain had completely collapsed to try to accommodate the mass. Amazingly, she had no symptoms beyond headaches, and her neurologic examination was completely normal. Meningiomas are almost always benign and so surgery would be curative. But without it, she would meet the same fate as Francky, dying when the pressure in her skull forced the brain downward, pinching off vital structures.

A forty-year-old pastor named Jean-Rémy had progressively lost vision in his right eye and then began to lose peripheral vision in his left eye. By the time we saw him, all he could see of the world was through the right half of his left eye. This pattern of visual loss suggested a tumor of the pituitary gland, which his CT scan confirmed. The tumor had grown so massive that it had extended from the gland's compartment at the base of the brain far upward into the brain itself. Without surgery, he would become blind and suffer severe complications of hormonal imbalances as his pituitary gland failed.

All of these patients could be big saves with neurosurgery. Their tumors were inside the skull but not within the brain itself, causing neurologic symptoms by compressing important structures rather than by invasion of healthy brain tissue.

I remembered when I had first heard about Janel's case from Martineau. It had struck me at the time as a unique instance in my two years working in Haiti when bringing a patient with a neurologic condition to the US would make a major difference. Part of the argument to our colleagues for bringing Janel to Boston had been that it wasn't likely to be a common request. After all, brain tumors account for only about one percent of all tumors, and some types of tumors within the brain itself were unlikely to be potential big saves even with surgery.

Then there was Francky, who could have been a big save. Now these three patients could be big saves. The CT scanner at HUM had opened Pandora's box: we were diagnosing more and more patients with conditions we couldn't treat.

This is something I was accustomed to in neurology since there are several neurological conditions that have no effective treatment— diseases like ALS and Alzheimer's disease. There's nothing more heartbreaking than telling patients that I know exactly what's causing their symptoms but have nothing to offer beyond helping them and their families come to terms with the diagnosis and prepare for an inevitable demise. Though I was comfortable diagnosing neurologic diseases that I couldn't treat in the US, the CT scanner at HUM was leading to the diagnosis of conditions that were treatable, just not in Haiti.

I wrote to Ian about these three new patients and sent him cell phone snapshots of their CT scans. I concluded the message:

> After everything that happened with Janel, I don't
> know if Brigham will be excited to do another charitable
> neurosurgical case. Any ideas of other avenues to explore
> to get these patients the care they need? They have much
> better baseline function than Janel—all ambulatory young to
> middle-aged adults with normal cognition.

Ian replied:

> I still think we should try to do these cases here. We will go
> nearly a lifetime without seeing another tumor like Janel's—
> and he was so debilitated before. These other cases sound
> like they will not require anywhere near the hospital length of
> stay that Janel required.

All of what he wrote was true. I could try to convince the hospital
that Janel's case had been an outlier in terms of medical, psychosocial,
and financial aspects. But would they believe me? Would they question
my judgment even if I told them this? After all, I had said Janel was
a college student who would walk into the hospital, have his surgery,
and walk out of the hospital. Nothing could have been further from
the truth, though I'd had no way of knowing that when I originally
proposed bringing him to Boston.

I had actually seen these three new patients with my own eyes. They
were very different from Janel, with minimal disability and a far lower
level of surgical complexity. But I had never explained to the hospital
administration that I hadn't actually seen Janel before we began the
process of advocating for his care. Perhaps it wouldn't have changed
anything if I had, but the conversation might have been different.

I worried that my enthusiasm to care for a patient as complex as Janel
could preclude us from caring for more straightforward neurosurgical
patients from Haiti at Brigham. In retrospect, I had led with a challenging, costly case. At the time, I had seen no choice, and I would likely
do the same thing again. But if I had known about all of these patients
from the outset, would I have strategized to bring a straightforward
patient first, ensuring a success and a good feeling for all involved to
pave the way for the next case? Or would I have felt Janel's case was the
most advanced and urgent? Maybe I would have just tried to bring all
of them, starting with whoever got their passport and visa first.

Despite my desire to help, I felt reluctant to try to bring another patient from Haiti to Boston for brain surgery. But it was pointless looking backward now. Just because Janel was back in the ICU after his fourth neurosurgery, why should that affect my approach to these new patients in front of us who needed our care? I had to try to do my best for all of them. I responded to Ian that I agreed we should go for it, and that we should begin working on cost estimates for these patients so we could see if Brigham would be willing to provide them with free care.

After the shunt removal and ETV, Janel remained unresponsive for days the way he had after his three prior surgeries. When he finally woke up, he didn't speak or interact at all and wasn't eating. Over the following days, he became progressively more sleepy and difficult to rouse. A CT scan showed his ventricles were beginning to balloon again.

Ian wrote to me while I was still in Haiti:

> Janel needs a shunt. He needs more CSF [cerebrospinal fluid] diversion than an ETV can provide. Sorry.

And so Janel went for neurosurgery number five.

I returned from Haiti to find Janel at his worst. He was lying in bed, motionless, unresponsive to voice, unresponsive to physical stimulation. A thick tan liquid ran from a pump into a small yellow tube entering his nose and snaking down into his stomach to try to give him some nutrition in anticipation of his upcoming chemotherapy.

A follow-up MRI showed that Janel's tumor was even smaller than on his last scan, meaning the radiation and chemotherapy had worked. But I was becoming increasingly concerned that although Janel's life may have been saved, the treatments had left him no better—and perhaps worse—than he had been before he came to

Boston for treatment. Saving his life without necessarily improving it was a risk we had all acknowledged from the outset. But looking at Janel, I couldn't help but think of the crude critique medical students sometimes make of neurosurgeons and neurologists: "Neurosurgeons make vegetables; neurologists water them." If Janel wasn't awake and couldn't eat on his own, I couldn't imagine putting him through more chemotherapy.

Feeling dejected, I left his room in the neuro-ICU. As I walked out, I saw one of my colleagues from neurology residency who was doing advanced training in neuro-oncology.

"Seeing your friend from Haiti . . ." she said with a forced half smile, her tone ambiguous as to whether she was asking me or simply stating a fact.

"Yeah," I sighed. "Are you involved in his care now?"

"I'm just following him from the neuro-oncology team while he's hospitalized," she said.

I nodded. "Thanks," I said.

"We should chat about him . . . I mean, he's not really . . ." She trailed off and glanced away.

"We're old friends. Tell me what you really think," I said, forcing a brief smile.

She looked down at her clogs. "I mean, I just met him this admission, but . . ." She looked up at me and paused. "Well, what are we doing here?" she said, softly but sternly. "He looks terrible. You're not really thinking of trying to give him more chemo, are you? I mean, I'm sure the oncologists would do it, but what's the goal here if he looks this bad?"

She stared at me, expressionless. I could tell the situation upset her. And I could imagine that neuro-oncology training had been trying for her, seeing patients die or become extremely disabled from aggressive brain tumors, with the tools of modern medicine often nearly powerless to make a major or lasting difference.

Now it was my turn to look down at my shoes. "Believe me, I'm asking myself the same questions," I said, shaking my head. "But at his best, he walks, he talks . . . he even sings and dances with the nurses . . . You're seeing him at his worst."

She raised her eyebrows cynically, cocking her head slightly to the side.

"I wouldn't believe it either if I were in your position, but it's true," I told her. "Look, he was completely unresponsive for nearly a month after the first surgeries, and I thought we'd wrecked him. But then one day he woke up, and a few weeks later he was walking. He's been through two seizures and two surgeries in the last week. We have to give him a chance to wake up more. He always takes a long time to come around after surgery."

Even as I said all this, I didn't feel optimistic. And she could easily perceive that.

"I guess we'll see," she said, shaking her head and walking past me into the room.

As I walked away down the hallway, I heard her begin trying to examine him. "Janel . . . Ja-nel! . . . Ja-*nel*!! . . . *Ja-nel!!!*"

Janel did wake up and eventually started eating on his own over the following week, but he had lost a lot of ground. Spending more than two weeks in bed after the seizures and surgeries, he had become too weak to stand on his own. We were unable to get free rehab for him again, and Hermide was understandably reluctant to take him home in such a disabled state. But we didn't have any other options, and she agreed to do it.

Janel spent most of his time at Hermide's asleep. When she brought him food, he could eat on his own, but otherwise he refused to get out of bed. After her previous experiences, she decided not to try to push him to do anything. She just let him sleep.

She did find, however, that he seemed happy to be taken to church on Sundays. One Sunday, she and the women who lived with her managed to get Janel into the car to take him to church. Moments after they had him seated in the pew, he began shaking and collapsed, hitting his chin on the floor. They called 911, and he was taken to a local hospital and then transferred to Brigham.

At Brigham, Janel immediately got a CT scan. Fortunately, it didn't show any problem with his shunt. But his blood tests showed low levels of his anti-seizure medication. When I told Hermide, she wasn't surprised.

"Well, he spits them out," she said shaking her head and making an exasperated clicking sound. "I didn't want to give him extra because I have no idea how much he swallows. I don't want to overdose him."

We switched him to a liquid form of the medicine—the one used for children—and sent him back home with Hermide. If she was unhappy about taking him home, she didn't say anything. But we were also afraid to ask. Where else would he go?

Janel's recent setbacks had put chemotherapy on hold until he was well enough to tolerate it. If anyone else on our team aside from me was wondering if he would ever be well enough, nobody mentioned it. But a few days later, Janel's oncologist broached the topic:

> I just wanted to revisit the idea of treating Janel. I still remain committed to his care, but I want to make sure we are doing right by him. I have serious concerns about further treatment for him, especially considering his poor functional status (Hermide per report can't get him to do anything). Chemotherapy would definitely drop his blood counts and set him up for further medical complications—and make him super sick. His course has been tenuous to date and his recovery from any event is delayed. His type of tumor is rare and we do not even know if adjuvant chemotherapy is necessary or not. There is evidence of residual disease on last MRI, although treatment to date may have been sufficient

to stabilize his disease for now. I recommend no further chemotherapy for now.

I will meet with Janel again before moving forward with chemotherapy but he has never been able to participate fully in a conversation with me and I have no confidence that he is giving me fully informed consent. I have always relied on Hermide and she thus far has wanted to remain aggressive.

I replied:

We had been wondering about the best way forward as well given his current status, and also felt that it is hard to know whether it would be appropriate to consider further treatment. Our hope had been that he would improve to his postsurgical baseline, which he appeared to be doing in the hospital, but it sounds as though overall he spends more time at his worst than at his best. I imagine if asked directly, his family and Hermide would want to do everything possible as you said, but I agree that it is not clear that this is what is best for him given how much suffering he would incur due to treatment, and for unclear gain. Presuming everyone agrees, I would lean against treating him at this stage and let him be comfortable with his family in Haiti.

Anne and Michelle agreed. So did Hermide. If our goal was to reduce Janel's suffering, it was hard to imagine keeping him in the US for six more months, sick and alone, at risk for complications of aggressive treatment with unknown benefit.

I had been reluctant to give up, but was it because of all he'd been through or because of all we'd been through? Probably some of both. Though I had no way of communicating with Janel, I suspected he'd be happier back in Haiti. Anne called Wilner in Haiti and explained that

Janel was too sick to get any further treatment. We began planning Janel's return home.

Since Janel had made so much progress in rehab at HUM during his last visit, we were hoping he could return there to try to regain some of the ground he had lost. He was worse now than when he had previously left Boston for rehab in Haiti, and we weren't even sure he could really participate in physical therapy, but it seemed worth a try.

The HUM rehab team was happy to work with him, but they wanted to know where he would go afterward. Martineau felt that Janel's mother's house was far too remote to be safe for Janel. If he had a seizure or any other medical complication, it would be nearly impossible to get him to a hospital—let alone a road to a hospital—quickly enough. Martineau was also concerned that Janel's mom would not be able to take care of Janel on her own, physically or financially.

Martineau asked Wilner if Janel could go back to staying with him, as he had for the year before Janel went to Boston. Unfortunately, Wilner told Martineau he no longer had space to take care of Janel.

We were in a difficult spot. We wanted to get Janel home, but there was no safe place for Janel to go home to.

"I guess we could cure his brain tumor, but we can't cure his poverty," I lamented to Michelle when we tried to come up with a plan.

"Right?!" She smiled sadly. "We're going to have to start thinking about relocating him and his mom to Mirebalais."

"We can do that?" I asked.

"I don't think we have much choice," she replied.

As we were thinking through all of this, an article I'd written about Janel many months earlier came out in a medical journal. It was a brief two-page essay in which I discussed some of the struggles we'd wrestled with trying to get Janel the care he needed, bridging the worlds of poverty-stricken rural Haiti and a high-tech academic hospital in Boston.

I wrote about the challenges we had faced presenting both the potential benefits and the potential risks of surgery in a place where hope is scarce and faith in medical miracles is strong. I reflected on how my colleagues in Haiti had helped me understand that I was misapplying my patient-centered US medical way of thinking in a place where many patients wanted doctors to decide what was right for them, not leave them with complex choices to decide on their own. I explored the objections we had encountered when we proposed pouring extensive resources into the care of a single individual and tried to tear them down in Paul Farmer–inspired arguments based on the first principles of doctoring:

> *In resource-limited settings, healthy debates center around*
> *hackneyed (but not entirely false) stereotypes that physicians focus*
> *on helping individual patients without always considering the larger*
> *system, while public health practitioners focus on the system without*
> *always accounting for how it will serve individual patients . . . In*
> *a case like this, traditional concepts of public health break down.*
> *A primary goal of global health is building capacity to raise the*
> *basic level of care and access to it. But in so doing, what happens*
> *to patients whose diagnoses are discovered by the new system, the*
> *new capacity, and the new access to it? Is it "sustainable" to turn a*
> *blind eye and focus on simpler problems first? When clinicians are*
> *faced with patients like this one, the theoretical principles of "cost-*
> *effectiveness" and "sustainability" seem tenuous alongside the simple*
> *tenets of the Hippocratic oath.*

Reading my words months later, they sounded naïve. How many times had I railed to friends and colleagues about those who criticized our caring for Janel as not being cost-effective or sustainable? But now I saw that I was equally worthy of critique. Had I really thought through the whole trajectory of what it meant to care for Janel, or had I just seen the medical problem and rushed in to try to fix it without thinking through the true cost of intervening in someone's health—and life—in this way? Had I really understood all that would need to be done to make this truly sustainable for Janel—a house, food, a source of income for him and his mom?

After the article's previous paragraph, one line followed:

On the other hand, what does it mean to "Do no harm" in a complex context that is not one's own place of practice?

In the article, I asked the question as a transition to discussing the challenges we faced explaining risk and benefit in a different culture. But now the question of whether we had done more harm than good loomed large. Had Janel's life been saved only to leave him in a state of disability so profound that he couldn't survive at home without completely restructuring his environment? And if his environment had to be changed so much to accommodate him—a new house in a new community—would he truly be going home? Would his mother want to be moved to a place where she knew nobody and had no social support? Would the new community accept her and Janel, and how would they react if they learned PIH was paying her bills and not theirs?

The article closed:

As our patient smilingly takes his first steps after a long recovery from two complex neurosurgeries and begins a treatment plan devised by a tumor board of world experts, we celebrate one small victory against inequity, against poverty, and against the odds. Yet we cannot lose sight of how many patients remain undiagnosed and untreated simply due to lack of access to basic—let alone specialized—health care. We brought this patient to modern medicine, but we must work tirelessly to bring modern medicine to all patients.

I remembered watching the cell phone video Michelle had made of the moment Janel smilingly took his first steps, and celebrating the milestone with Martineau as we watched it in Haiti. But by the time the article came out, Janel was bedbound and mute. It was unclear if we could safely get him home to Haiti. The article felt insincere. Janel was no longer smiling, no longer walking, and his uncertain future hardly felt like a victory. I believed in the concluding sentiment, but I wondered if I really had the knowledge, skills, or experience to carry it out effectively. Who was I to swoop in and try to do what I thought was the right thing if I didn't really know the right way to do it? Was there even a right way?

Despite feeling uncomfortable that the article had inadvertently sugarcoated the story since the situation had changed so much since I had written it, I decided I should send it to all those who had helped. I emailed it to my colleagues with both a thanks and an apology:

> I wanted to share with you this article I wrote about Janel that came out today. Although the paper was submitted a long time ago and his subsequent progress has not quite continued on the same high note on which the end of his story is told here, hopefully this article can raise the awareness and support necessary to help patients like Janel in Haiti and elsewhere much earlier in their disease course in the future.

I received some solace in a reply from Père Eddy, the priest and psychologist who runs the HUM mental health team:

> Whatever happens after, Janel will remain an icon of hope for the multitude of the vulnerable people over the world. Our hands can touch theirs and the human chain will never break!

His moving words reminded me of the advice I had received from another colleague in Haiti when I had agonized over the potential unintended negative consequences if we tried to care for Janel and something went wrong. She had suggested I also consider the potential unintended positive consequences of trying to help a patient in a place where many die of treatable diseases or become progressively disabled with no hope for recovery simply due to lack of access to healthcare. If the patient does well, she had said, it could give hope to his entire community. Even if he doesn't do well—which would certainly happen eventually if he stayed in Haiti with no care—the solidarity demonstrated by trying to help him could still have a positive impact, giving hope where hope is hard to come by.

I was beginning to realize that maybe this was just how it feels to do this work. Proceed on principle, struggle to a solution, address obstacles as they arise. Even knowing what I knew at that point, I couldn't imagine having simply left Janel to suffer because of unforeseeable or even foreseeable challenges. If we frame problems in terms of their constraints rather than their possibilities, prioritizing risk avoidance above all else, we are less motivated to find solutions. In Janel's case, we would have given up at the first accusation that trying to care for him was too costly, too impractical, and had too many potential negative outcomes.

Talking with one of my colleagues, I expressed how bad I felt about the way things had turned out for Janel and how I struggled with the feeling that we'd only made things worse by intervening.

"You had to try," she responded compassionately but firmly. "We do this all the time in medicine—accept the risks hoping for the benefits. Sometimes we succeed, but sometimes the disease wins. You couldn't just give up without trying, and the patient and his family so very much wanted you to try. You guys did so much for him."

In spite of all of the challenges with Janel, I was already beginning the process of advocating for the three patients with brain tumors I had met on my last trip to Haiti to come to Brigham. But what lessons should I take from Janel's case as we tried again with these new patients?

I wasn't sure.

———————

Janel ended up back in the hospital at Brigham. Hermide had come to wake him up and found his bed empty. Janel was on the floor next to it. He had urinated on himself and was unresponsive. We presumed he'd had an unwitnessed seizure and that Hermide had found him in the confused state that often follows a seizure. But when he arrived at Brigham and we checked the blood level of his anti-seizure medication, it was actually elevated far above the therapeutic range. The medication level had become so high that he'd suffered toxicity from it and fallen unconscious. After he was in the hospital for a few days off the medication, the drug level fell to the appropriate range again, and he woke up.

One of our epilepsy specialist colleagues told us that the liquid form of the medication that we'd given him since he was spitting out the pills could sometimes get concentrated at the bottom of the container, leading to toxic levels of the medicine. We switched him back to the pill form (the liquid wouldn't be available in Haiti anyway) and sent him back to Hermide's with a plan for some follow-up appointments and repeat labs in the coming weeks.

Janel languished at Hermide's. He slept twenty hours a day. He refused to go from his bed into a chair. He ate little and sometimes fell asleep while eating. He began losing weight. In medical terminology, he developed what we call "failure to thrive." The term always seemed to me to be an odd attempt to spin a tragic condition positively, since patients labeled with "failure to thrive" were so far from anything that could be considered thriving. Janel was not only failing to "thrive" but failing to perform even basic functions beyond sleeping.

We told the rehab team at HUM that PIH was working on housing but we couldn't wait for it to be in place before Janel's return to Haiti to begin rehab, and they agreed to take him.

By the time Janel had completed his follow-up appointments and a bed was ready on the rehab ward at HUM, it was mid-December. Hermide offered to travel back to Haiti with him so she could stay there for Christmas. Nearly one year after Janel had first arrived in Boston, he was finally going back to Haiti.

I wondered what we had achieved for him with two trips to Boston, five surgeries, and six weeks of chemotherapy and radiation. He no longer had a brain tumor, but now he had a shunt and a seizure disorder and had presumably suffered some degree of psychological distress. There was no clear plan for where he would live when he got home.

So much for walking out of the hospital, so much for a big save.

13

think we should start a neurology residency here," said Dr. Kerling Israel, the director of medical education for the entire PIH/ZL network in Haiti. We were sitting at a small circular table in her office in the upstairs administration area of HUM, the pages of our open notebooks fluttering each time the circulating desk fan rotated past them.

I raised my eyebrows and looked at her. "That would be . . ." I wasn't sure how to complete the sentence: ambitious, challenging, crazy, or . . . the culmination of our neurology work in Haiti for the preceding three years.

When I first became interested in global health, I wondered if there was any role for a neurologist in the field. All of the big names in global health, like Paul Farmer, seemed to be infectious disease specialists, and all of the big funding seemed to go to programs to fight HIV, tuberculosis, and malaria. Otherwise, it seemed like there was work for surgical teams who could do a large number of surgeries in a brief international visit—such as cleft palate repairs or cataract surgeries—and then have the patients follow up with their local providers. But neurology? Neurology requires long-term care of patients, so it's not suitable to this mission-type model. And I had read that life expectancy is much lower in poor countries compared to rich countries—did people live long enough to develop common neurologic diseases like stroke, Parkinson's disease, and dementia?

Then I learned that stroke is the second leading cause of death and disability worldwide, disproportionately affecting people in low- and

middle-income countries. I discovered that the large majority of patients with epilepsy live in poorer regions of the world, many remaining untreated due to lack of access to a neurologist. And despite this
enormous burden of neurologic disease in the poorest parts of the
world, the average number of neurologists in low-income countries is
about three per ten million population, one hundred times lower than
in high-income countries like the US. And that's just the average. Many
low-income countries have no neurologists at all.

When I first met Michelle at Brigham and asked her how I could
help PIH as a neurologist, she replied instantly, "Come and teach our
doctors in Haiti." Not only were most patients unable to access the one
practicing neurologist in Haiti, who had fallen ill, but the general doctors these patients saw had never had access to a neurologist to learn
how to diagnose and treat neurologic conditions.

Michelle and Kerling thought that teaching neurology for a few
weeks each year would ideally have a greater impact on patient care
over the long term than seeing large numbers of patients for a few weeks
each year in a mission-type model. My colleagues in Haiti seemed to
enjoy having a neurologist give lectures and advise them on patients a
few times per year, and I found it meaningful too. But after two years,
I had started to wonder how much impact it was really having. On any
given trip, I would teach in two different hospitals, seeing patients with
different doctors all over each of these hospitals—internists, emergency room doctors, surgeons, psychologists. I felt that my teaching
efforts were spread thin.

"Pise gaye pa kime," laughed one of my colleagues in Haiti when I
explained my concern to him. It was a proverb I hadn't heard before:
Pissing all over the place makes no bubbles.

"Chyen gen kat pa, men li pa ka kouri nan kat chemen," said another.
Another new proverb for my collection: A dog has four legs, but it can't
run on four paths at once.

It was this feeling of being spread thin that had led me to focus my
efforts on providing neurology training for Martineau and the internal

medicine residents at HUM. Over the course of the previous year we had seen more than 150 patients together. Martineau and the residents I worked with became quite skilled at neurologic diagnosis and treatment. My colleagues in the HUM leadership, like Kerling, thought the program had been a success.

If such narrowing of focus could improve neurology education and patient care in Haiti, how far and deep could we go if our team devoted all of our efforts to an even smaller cohort all year for several years? Yes, a neurology residency would be the culmination of our work in Haiti. If we could train several Haitian doctors as neurologists in the coming years, and then they could train the next generation of neurologists, we would be creating something truly self-sustaining. In the field, it's what we call "mentoring ourselves out of our roles."

HUM had just launched Haiti's first emergency medicine residency program, directed and staffed by visiting US-based emergency medicine faculty who spent weeks at a time as clinician-educators supervising local physician trainees as they cared for patients in the emergency room. They had dozens of visiting faculty to make sure that every day and night shift was covered for the entire year. In contrast, I was the only neurologist working with PIH, and I had only eight weeks free from Brigham each year to spend in Haiti.

"It would be amazing to think about a neurology residency here modeled after the emergency medicine program," I said to Kerling, "but I'm just one person." I smiled apologetically.

Kerling smiled back politely. Then she looked at me seriously. "We should start thinking about it. It's the next logical step."

Kerling is ambitious. Under her leadership, HUM established itself as a trailblazer in Haitian medical education. Over the preceding three years, HUM had initiated not only the unique emergency medicine program but also residency programs in internal medicine, pediatrics, surgery, and obstetrics-gynecology, all of which were the first residency programs outside a major city in Haiti.

"How much time can you spend here next year?" she asked.

"At least eight weeks, like this year," I said. "Maybe I could try to ask for a little more time." I imagined I could probably negotiate a few more weeks away from Brigham for the first one or two years if we were trying to get a neurology residency off the ground at HUM. But even if I could somehow spend half of each year in Haiti, I was concerned it still wouldn't provide the continuity of training necessary to make the program successful. I told Kerling I would think more about it.

As I thought it through, I wondered what it would be like to move to Haiti for a few years at the start of the program. I envied my colleagues who had the opportunity to live and work in rural Haiti or other similar settings for years at a time. They had a unique understanding of the places where they worked. They had mastered the local language and understood nuances of local culture. And I thought they had a better sense than short-term visitors like me of what local life was really like, at least to the extent that a foreign visitor could. Maybe the moment had arrived for me to move to Haiti.

Nina was supportive of the possibility of me relocating for a year or two. Despite seeming worlds away, Haiti was only four and a half hours from Boston via one of the direct flights JetBlue had started running each week, so it wouldn't be hard to come home for a few days here and there. But I had just begun a very fulfilling job at Brigham and had been asked to take on some teaching roles at Harvard Medical School. I worried that if I disappeared for a year or two it would be hard to pick up where I'd left off when I returned.

The next time I saw Michelle she told me she had good news. A neurologist had emailed PIH out of the blue asking if he could volunteer in Haiti. When I spoke with him, he said he had no prior experience in a setting like Haiti, but he seemed enthusiastic and thoughtful. And he had a position that allowed him twelve weeks away each year. If I could negotiate a similar amount of time in Haiti, together we could cover almost half the calendar year. If we gave the neurology trainees in Haiti a monthlong rotation in Boston at Brigham, a month of vacation, and accounted for the Christmas, Easter, All Saints', and Carnival holidays, when few patients come to the hospital and clinics are closed, twenty-four weeks would provide on-the-ground coverage for more than half the academic year.

Still, it seemed inadequate. If we were going to ensure the success of a new program and rigorous training for its first residents, I thought we should have continuous coverage for at least the first two years.

I set up a conference call with Kerling and Michelle. I told them we had made some progress by finding a second neurologist willing to commit a surprisingly significant number of weeks to working in Haiti, but I thought it would take more time to build a bigger team.

"Should we aim for a year from now?" I asked them.

"No," Kerling said. "Twenty-four weeks of coverage is plenty. I think we should start in the fall."

"But it will leave so many open weeks," I said, concerned.

"To you it doesn't seem like enough," Kerling replied, "but right now we have next to nothing in neurology. So the first step is to have something. Then it could grow from there."

I didn't like the idea of starting a program with patchy coverage. It would be suboptimal for the first resident to be left unsupervised for weeks at a time, and hard to address any inevitable issues from afar. But this line of argument wasn't getting me anywhere. I tried a different approach.

"I'm just one year out of my own residency," I said and laughed. "I'm so junior. Should I really be in charge of running a program at this stage? Maybe we should wait another year or two."

"I don't know of any other neurologist who is going to do this if you don't," Michelle said.

"Okay, but shouldn't we at least wait until I have some more experience?" I asked.

"I'm not sure I know of any neurologists with more experience in Haiti than you," Michelle replied.

"And we know you," Kerling added. "And you know us. You are the right person for the job."

"I agree we should try to do it," I said, "but I just think we should take some time to build a bigger team of faculty and think through some of the logistics. Maybe we wait one more year?"

"Once you start, people will see what you're doing," Kerling said, "and then I'm sure more neurologists will want to get involved. But we shouldn't wait for that. Let's go for it! It will evolve."

I sensed that they felt I was being too cautious. I suppose if everyone had waited for every detail to be in place to launch an enormous project like constructing HUM, perhaps it never would have happened. But for something much smaller in scale like training one neurologist over two years, I thought we should try to have more structure and staff in place before moving forward. Was I falling victim to what Paul Farmer would call a failure of imagination?

"Don't let perfect be the enemy of good," Michelle said, as if reading my thoughts.

I had one last concern. It was going to be an election year in Haiti. This would mean large and sometimes violent protests that could limit travel to and through the country. During the previous election cycle's violence several years prior, PIH had nearly needed to evacuate all of its Haiti-based employees.

I thought back to the night before leaving Boston on my second trip to Haiti a few years earlier. I had packed my backpack and put it next to the front door. I had set my email away message and signed over my Brigham pager. I was just about to go to sleep when I got a text message from one of my colleagues in Haiti:

> Massive protests planned for tomorrow. Not safe to travel in-country: road blocks, demonstrations, tear gas, etc.
> Re-book flight for next day.

I didn't sleep well that night. What if nobody had remembered to send me that message and I had shown up in Haiti? Could I have been caught up in the violence en route to Mirebalais? Would I have been stranded at the airport with no drivers safely able to come pick me up? How was it so unsafe that I could not travel one day but would be okay to travel the following day? I postponed my trip a week. Was this what I had to look forward to in a career in global health—danger, cancelled trips, uncertainty? Was I really cut out for this?

The trip ultimately went fine, as have all subsequent ones.

"Isn't it an election year next year?" I asked Kerling and Michelle. "Maybe it's not the best year to start a new program if we risk having trips cancelled and other disruptions."

Michelle and Kerling laughed gently. "The election year might be challenging," Michelle said. "But depending on what happens in the election, the year after might be even worse."

"You never know in Haiti," Kerling agreed. "So we can't think like that. When we have the opportunity here we have to proceed. If we keep postponing, waiting for stability . . . Well, stability may never come. But we still have to keep moving forward."

It looked like they weren't going to take no for an answer. So we agreed to launch a neurology residency program at HUM a few months later, starting small with just one resident at a time.

I negotiated with Brigham for a few more weeks in Haiti for that year and recruited some of my colleagues to volunteer for a week or two. Meanwhile, HUM put out a call for applicants and invited the most promising candidates to HUM for an exam and interview. They offered the first position to the top applicant, Dr. François Roosevelt, an internal medicine doctor in his late forties who had been in practice for nearly two decades. He had always wanted to get further training in a specialty, but no medical specialty training programs existed in Haiti. Our neurology program would be the first. And François would become the first Haitian neurologist to be trained in Haiti.

One of the first patients François and I evaluated together at HUM was a little boy named Davidson, who had been admitted to the pediatric ward. Davidson's faded light green hospital gown covered all but his head and arms. The gown was nearly the same color as the off-white sheets beneath him, making his cherubic face look like a small island floating in the ocean of his large hospital bed. He looked around curiously through calm, big eyes that framed a small, bridgeless button nose. Aside from his eyes, he didn't move any other part of his body.

Davidson's father, Enel, sat by his bedside in a dark green T-shirt. He stood slowly as we approached, appearing concerned but calm. He gently placed the black hardcover book he had been reading on the chair he had been sitting on. I glanced over at the book. BIB LA was engraved in gold block letters on its cover—a Haitian Creole translation of the Bible. Enel was small-framed with a strong build. His big eyes and prominent, high cheekbones gave his face an innocent, gentle, almost deer-like quality. He couldn't have been much older than early thirties and looked even younger.

Enel told us that Davidson was five years old and had developed normally until about age two, including being able to walk. Over the subsequent three years, he had become progressively paralyzed in both legs and then both arms, leaving him quadriplegic. Enel and Davidson lived in Port-de-Paix at the northern tip of Haiti, about an eight-hour drive from HUM. Enel had traveled all over the country with his son by bus and *taptap*, trying to find someone who could help them. Someone had told him that Davidson needed a CT scan and could get one for free at HUM, where he might also encounter a neurologist who occasionally visited from *lòt bò a*—the other side.

As François and I approached Davidson's bed to examine him, the small boy watched calmly, following us with his eyes without turning his head. He could tell us his name and count to ten. With great effort, he could just barely move his left arm back and forth on the bed, but his right arm and both legs were completely paralyzed. All of his limbs were extremely stiff when we tried to bend them—spasticity. With even the slightest tap of François's reflex hammer on Davidson's elbow creases or knees, the boy's limbs shot lightning-fast off the bed—hyperreflexia. When François gently scratched the bottom of each of Davidson's feet with the tip of his reflex hammer, Davidson's big toes rose like a thumbs-up, and his other toes fanned apart—a Babinski sign.

François looked up at me and smiled. "Spinal cord!" he exclaimed enthusiastically, proud of his newly acquired neurologic diagnostic skills.

"Exactly," I replied, smiling back at him. "The combination of spastic quadriplegia, hyperreflexia, and bilateral Babinski signs with no problems above the neck suggests a problem in the cervical spinal cord. Now, in my experience in Haiti, non-traumatic paraplegia or quadriplegia is either Pott's or it's not."

Pott's disease is a tuberculosis infection of the spine that causes one or more of the vertebrae to collapse, which can lead to compression of the spinal cord. Tuberculosis (TB) is mistakenly considered a disease of the past by people who live in high-income countries, where it is exceedingly rare. But TB isn't a disease of the past in the world's poorest countries, where it continues to infect ten million people per year and kill more than one million people per year—more than AIDS. Haiti has the highest yearly rate of new tuberculosis cases in the Western Hemisphere.

"Let's feel for any spinal deformity that would suggest a collapsed vertebra due to Pott's," I said to François.

As my hand approached Davidson's neck, his eyes grew wider. And as I pushed on the bones of his cervical spine in the back of his neck, he grimaced in pain. "Sorry, sorry, almost done," I said as I quickly walked my fingertips up and down his neck. Nothing felt out of the ordinary. I gently tried to bring his chin to his chest, but it was immovable, completely rigid. He started to cry softly, big warm tears streaming down his cheeks. "Okay, done. Sorry. I'm done now. Sorry."

Enel wiped Davidson's tears with his hospital gown while François and I stepped away to talk through his case.

"I don't feel anything to suggest Pott's," I said, "but we still might see a bony defect on an x-ray or CT scan that could help us make the diagnosis."

We sat down at the nearby nurses' station to review Davidson's CT scan on a computer. The scan didn't show any problem with the bones of the spine, so Pott's was off the list. I worried this meant we were very unlikely to make a diagnosis for this young boy. We had seen so many paralyzed patients with no diagnosis in Haiti that we had developed a name for the scenario: cryptogenic paraplegia (or quadriplegia)—paralysis of both legs (or all four limbs) of cryptic origin.

But Davidson's case turned out not to be cryptogenic at all. At the point where his spinal cord arose from the base of the brain, his CT scan revealed a huge cyst compressing the spinal cord to the width of a thin string.

No wonder he kept his neck rigid and refused to move it. He was literally hanging on by a thread—a thread of spinal cord connecting his head to his body. Any further compression, perhaps even if he bent his neck the wrong way, could cut off the brain's signals to his lungs to breathe. His neck muscles must have become rigid over time from not moving in order to guard his spinal cord.

It was hard to tell if the abnormality on Davidson's CT scan was in the spinal cord itself or just compressing it from the outside. If it was just compression, maybe surgery could relieve the pressure and give him some of his motor function back. On the other hand, his spinal cord could be irreversibly damaged from three years of being so severely deformed.

Here we go again, I thought. In any rich country, this unfortunate child wouldn't have had to wait three years for a diagnosis, let alone the diagnosis of a problem that might have been fixable before it got to this point. But if whatever this was kept growing, it could eventually affect his breathing. He would suffocate and die.

Should I try to get Davidson to the US for surgery? Removing the cyst might do nothing more than save him in this quadriplegic state, leading to a life of complete dependence on others. This would be a challenging existence anywhere in the world, but especially in a place like Haiti. Davidson would not have a power wheelchair that he could control with what little strength remained in his left hand. And even if he did, navigating the rocky, hilly dirt roads would be treacherous. There would be no accessible ramps to enter schools, which in any case would have no adaptive technology to help him learn in his paralyzed state. If his father died, he'd have no way to take care of himself. He would be as bad off as Janel—maybe even worse. At least Janel could move a little.

I looked over at this small boy in his big bed. His eyes were filled with intelligence as he scanned the room, calmly observing his surroundings. He was in a corner bed, the exact same spot in the adult ward where Francky had died a few months earlier. Wincing, I looked away, closed my eyes, and shook my head. The possibility of getting involved in another potentially tragic story seemed overwhelming. I felt like I had failed Francky, who had died with false hope that we would be able to help him. I had managed to get Janel to the US, but nothing had gone as planned and I wasn't sure we had really helped him in the end. It was probably just too late in his case. It might already be too late for Davidson too.

As I began to feel depressed by the deep hopelessness of it all, I realized I was going have to make a strong effort not to let my past failures overinfluence how I approached this boy's care. To start, I needed an expert opinion from a pediatric neurosurgeon to get a sense of whether there was any way to help Davidson. If there wasn't, at least I could be straightforward with his father about this devastating prognosis. If it looked like surgery could help him . . . I decided I would cross that bridge when I came to it.

I Googled pediatric neurosurgeons specialized in spine surgery in Boston and found Dr. Mark Proctor, the chair of neurosurgery at Boston Children's Hospital, which is just across the street from us at Brigham. I dashed off an email to him about Davidson's case.

While I awaited Mark's reply, François and I explained to Enel that the scan showed a problem at the top of his son's spinal cord. We weren't sure what it was. Whatever it might be, there was no treatment for it in Haiti. It was possible surgery might help, but we weren't sure. And even if surgery could help, it couldn't be done in Haiti, and we couldn't promise we could get him to the US due to the complexities of costs and visas. Would he like us to look into that possibility further? Yes. Did they have means to afford surgery abroad? No. Did they have passports? No. We told him we would try to get a better understanding of what might be possible after consulting with some colleagues in the US.

Just as Ian had wanted an MRI to better understand Janel's case before committing to surgery, Mark wrote back that he needed an MRI for Davidson before he could say whether he thought he could help him. I was headed home to Boston, but Martineau offered to help arrange this.

A few weeks later we received the MRI report, which confirmed our impression from the CT: there was a large cystic mass compressing the spinal cord. But it was unclear what it was. A tumor? A congenital malformation that hadn't become symptomatic until early childhood? An infectious cyst from some type of parasite? I took screenshots of the key images and emailed them to Mark. A few moments later I received his surgically brief reply:

> Really bizarre. Not sure what it is, but it seems like something that could be treated and afford the child great benefit. I would definitely like to proceed. We can use neurosurgery free care pool.

I began excitedly texting Anne that Davidson's case was accepted for free care and that I looked forward to working together again. But then I remembered that an initial yes had been just the beginning of a months-long saga to obtain Janel's passport. Since Martineau no longer had his government connections to help us, Enel and Davidson would need to go through the process on their own.

A month went by. And then two. Enel's passport finally came through, but he was still waiting for Davidson's.

In the meantime, Anne arranged free housing for Davidson and Enel at the Ronald McDonald House around the corner from Boston Children's for when they would arrive. Another month passed. And then another two. Still no passport for Davidson.

When I wrote to update Mark and the Boston Children's team that we were still waiting for the patient's passport to come through, they replied that if surgery was not scheduled within two months, they would lose their free-care allotment from the hospital for the fiscal year. They told us that they had been unable to offer free neurosurgery to another child because of their commitment to our patient's care. If we couldn't get Davidson to Boston for surgery in time, their free-care allotment for the year would go to waste.

I felt horrible. Another child had missed out, and Davidson could miss out too, all due to administrative delays in Haiti. Not only was this bad for the patients, but it would also reflect poorly on us for any future efforts to bring a patient to Boston Children's. After all of the twists and turns of Janel's care—not to mention his unfortunate outcome—I was worried we could be giving ourselves a "strike two" in our attempts to create a pathway for big save neurosurgical cases to come to Boston from Haiti.

We decided to ask one of our colleagues in Haiti to interface with Enel to try to help him navigate the passport process to get Davidson to Boston in time. Unfortunately, our colleague came back with bad news:

> Enel told me, YESTERDAY, that he has/had a passport.
> Passport agency took it to use for Davidson and lost it
> apparently. They could not find it . . . *tèt chaje*!

Tèt chaje literally means "burdened head." It's one of many expressions describing one's head in Haitian Creole, along with *tèt cho* ("hot head"—angry and/or disorganized), *tèt anba* ("head down"—embarrassed or passive), *tèt vid* ("empty head"—out of it), *tèt gwo* ("big head"—anxious), and *tèt lou* ("heavy head"—worried). *Tèt chaje* is a common expression of bewilderment, frustration, and/or disgust in Haiti, something like "Oh my God!" in English. How could a government agency lose one of its citizen's passports? Sadly, in Haiti, it wasn't so unbelievable.

Our colleague in Haiti wrote to us again a few days later to let us know that Davidson's passport had come through, but Enel's was still missing.

Since we were cutting it close, I wondered about just bringing Davidson to Boston and looking for a host family. Bringing Janel alone had had its challenges, to say the least. Would it be simpler for a five-year-old than it had been for a twenty-three-year-old? More challenging? A five-year-old alone in a hospital in a foreign country was certainly a suboptimal psychosocial situation. But so was becoming progressively quadriplegic from an operable lesion due to a bureaucratic mess in Haiti when there was the possibility of free care just a short flight away. I called Anne to ask her thoughts.

Anne didn't know of any cases in which PIH had brought a child so young to the US without a relative. She thought she could convince her parents to house Davidson after his surgery, but she pointed out that the hospital was not likely to be amenable. Who would sign consent? Who would stay with the child overnight and help him communicate his needs to the staff?

We tried to call Enel to discuss this with him but were unable to reach him. Our local colleagues couldn't get in touch with him either.

The window for free care for Davidson was about to close.

I was headed back down to Haiti and offered to help with the passport situation if I could. But we were running out of time.

Tèt chaje!

14

The rehabilitation ward at HUM is a small, L-shaped white building with a bright orange door. One segment of the L has a gymnasium for physical therapy, the other, a small ward. The white interior walls are decorated with purple curtains, brightly colored tile mosaics, and posters of Haitian Creole proverbs:

Piti piti, zwazo fè nich li.
(Little by little, the bird builds its nest.)

Men anpil chay pa lou.
(Many hands make the burden lighter.)

Tout moun se moun.
(Every person is a person.)

Toutan tèt ou poko koupe espere met chapo.
(As long as your head is not cut off, you
still have hope to wear your hat.)

As I entered the rehab ward, I saw Janel lying in the last bed at the end on the right, past a young man with paraplegia (both legs paralyzed) from spine trauma, an elderly lady with hemiplegia (one side of the body paralyzed) from a stroke, and a teenage boy with severe mental and physical disabilities since childhood who'd been abandoned on

HUM's doorstep and had lived there ever since. Janel's hair had grown back thick and was matted in places. His mustache had grown out into a few long spindly whiskers at the edges. Even from across the ward, I could see the broad whites of his eyes, his familiar wide-eyed stare. He lay there, still.

Next to him was a thin older woman sitting in a chair, holding his hand. I realized immediately that she must be his mother. Her skin was darker than Janel's, her face showed the weathering of age with deep creases across her forehead and along each side of her mouth, and of course her eyes did not appear to bulge as Janel's did, but the resemblance was otherwise unmistakable. From beneath her bandana's swirling pattern of yellow, green, orange, and blue, a few short gray braids of hair peeked out, dangling in front of her ears. She wore a small blue, black, and yellow striped polo shirt and a black knee-length skirt that hung limply on her thin frame.

I paused. I had seen her briefly when she brought Janel to HUM over a year prior, but we hadn't spoken. Since then, my colleagues and I had taken her son for most of a year. She didn't have a phone, and so we were never able to talk directly to her. Wilner had assured us he visited her and updated her, but did she know of all of the setbacks, fluctuations, and behavioral outbursts? Had she shared the fear we'd had when he took weeks to wake up after surgery? Or had she been largely shielded from all of this by Wilner, just being told periodically that Janel was doing okay? I didn't really know what she knew. If she had hoped Janel would return from *lòt bò a*—the other side—miraculously cured, I imagined she must have been devastated by the failure of that hope to materialize. I thought of how disappointed she must be that he looked more or less the same as before he left—if not worse—sleeping his days away and minimally interactive when he was awake.

My Creole was coming along, but it wasn't good enough to explain that I was sorry he wasn't better, sorry he might even be worse. How would I apologize for any false hope we may have given her that he'd be saved or at least better than before?

I took a deep breath and made my way across the small ward between the two rows of hospital beds. As I approached Janel's mother,
she looked up at me with curiosity. Then she suddenly leapt up, her eyes
brightening as she smiled the same smile Janel had rarely revealed to
us, one so broad that it seemed to show every last tooth. She was missing many of her teeth, and many of those she did have were chipped or
crooked, but this didn't diminish the radiance of her smile. She spread
her long, thin arms outward as if preparing to embrace her own son.

"*Oo oo! Doktè! Doktè!*" she nearly sang, her voice high-pitched and
lilting. She hugged me close to her and moved her head from over one
of my shoulders to over the other, back and forth several times. She
continued to hug me, rocking us back and forth. "*Oo! Bondye ap beni
w! Apre Bondye se doktè! Oo-eee!*" she cried out. ("Oo! God bless you!
After God is the doctor! Oo-eee!")

I glanced over her shoulder at Janel. He looked the same as when
I had last seen him in Boston a few months prior. Mute, motionless,
staring blankly ahead. He still looked terrible. I was confused by his
mother's effusiveness.

"*Kouman Janel ye?*" I asked her tentatively. ("How is Janel?")

"*Li la!*" she exclaimed joyfully, releasing me and taking hold of my
hands, still smiling broadly. ("He's here!") "*Li byen, grace à Dye! Janel!
Salye doktè!*" ("He's good, thanks to God! Janel! Say hi to the doctor!")

There was no reaction from Janel.

This was *byen* (good)? She motioned excitedly for me to sit down in
the chair she had been sitting on. I tried to encourage her to sit there,
but she insisted. I was touched by her greeting but struggled to make
sense of how she could be so happy with him still looking so bad.

Then I thought of the first thing she had said: *Li la*—He's here.

In Haiti, saying "*Mwen la*" ("I'm here") is a common response when
people are asked, "How are you?" Although "I'm here" may sound
like the bare minimum of how one can be, it's actually a more positive response than some of the other frequent answers to the question, like "*M pa pi mal*" ("I'm not too bad") or "*N'ap kenbe*" ("We're

holding on"), not to mention "*N'ap lite*" ("We're struggling") or "*N'ap boule*" ("We're burning"). A colleague of mine in Haiti says they all essentially mean "I'm okay," but I've always been struck by the literal translations.

Li la—he's here. Janel was here, he was alive. Maybe that already exceeded his mother's expectations—in a place like Haiti, where so many people die of much more mundane and trivial causes than brain tumors, mere survival could be a gift. I remembered how months earlier I had agonized over whether Janel and his mother truly understood the risks of brain surgery in Boston, but they had been willing to do anything that had a chance of helping him. Though I'd felt defeated about how poorly Janel had done after all of modern medicine's attempts to save him, his mother was thrilled just to have him alive. What had seemed a tragic disappointment to me appeared to be a triumphant victory for her.

Deeply moved by Janel's mother's gratitude in spite of the outcome, I thought about how success and failure in medicine are never as sharply defined as we may think. That night, I wrote to one of my oncology colleagues:

> Not a spectacular outcome by any means from our perspective, but his mom was so happy and grateful for him being cared for. I suppose it's all relative in a place where so many people just seem to die for no reason. It really put the whole thing in perspective for me.

She replied:

> I guess it's not a huge victory, but in my neuro-oncology world, he's alive and home and well overall, which is about as good as you could hope for.

Midway through my week at HUM, I got an email from our local PIH/ZL administrative colleague who had been trying to help Enel with his passport. She wrote:

> Morning Aaron and Anne, I prayed last night—harder than usual—LOL and this morning, I was able to "find" Enel. He's in Port de Paix. I asked him to come asap. We spoke of having someone else travel with Davidson if he can't and he's ok with that. He's hoping to arrive in Mirebalais on Saturday so we can make a plan.

That weekend, while I was eating some rice and beans and reading an article on my phone in the staff house dining room by myself, I saw a man walk by the entrance to the house out of the corner of my eye. Could it have been Enel? He was supposed to come to Mirebalais at some point over the weekend. I didn't get a good look at him, and lots of people who stay or work in the house are constantly coming and going. A little boy ran after the man. *I guess not*, I thought. If it had been Enel, he would have been carrying his son since Davidson couldn't move. I went back to my lunch and article.

The man came into the dining room doorway and looked at me.

"*Doktè Aaron?*" he asked.

"*Monsieur Enel?*" I asked him.

We smiled and shook hands.

The little boy I had seen ran up behind him, grabbed onto his leg, peered curiously around it, and then flashed a big smile.

"*Se frè Davidson?*" I asked, smiling down at the little boy. ("Is this Davidson's brother?") He looked a lot like Davidson. But he didn't have the same cherubic cheeks I remembered from when I'd met him six months prior. And he could move.

"*No, li se Davidson,*" Enel replied calmly. ("No, that's Davidson.")

My smile faded abruptly. I must have misunderstood the Creole.

Davidson was bedbound and immobile, and this little boy had already scampered off while I tried to make sense of what Enel had just said.

"Li se Davidson?" I asked, eyebrows raised nearly to my hairline. ("That's Davidson?")

"Wi," Enel replied nonchalantly. ("Yes.")

"Li ka mache?!" I asked, bewildered. ("He can walk?!")

"Wi, li ka mache kounyea," Enel said casually and smiled softly. ("Yes, he can walk now.") He didn't seem fazed by my shocked confusion. I invited him to sit with me at the dining room table. Someone had brought a pizza from Port-au-Prince, and I cut him a slice. I sat down across from him at the table.

Davidson ran into the room, hopped up onto a chair at the table next to his dad, bent his legs under him, sat down on his feet, and looked eagerly at the pizza.

"Kouman li ka mache?" I asked Enel, unable to take my eyes off Davidson. ("How can he walk?")

"A few months ago he started to crawl," he said, cutting a piece of pizza for Davidson and putting it on his plate. "Then he started to walk." He took a bite of his slice of pizza, chewed it, and swallowed. "And now he can even run."

I was astonished. How could this be the same boy who just a few months ago was completely paralyzed from the neck down, crying in pain when we touched his neck?

"I didn't recognize him," I said.

"Yes," Enel explained, "since he became active again, he lost some weight."

I kept staring at Davidson. "Before he starts eating, can I examine him?" I asked.

Enel asked Davidson to put down his slice of pizza. He did so calmly, and I walked around the table to where he sat. I put my hands under his armpits, lifted him up, and sat him on the dining room table.

I tested his strength by having him pull and push my hands with his arms and legs—completely normal. I jiggled his arms and legs to test his tone—all were loose, the spasticity gone. I stiffened my first two fingers and tapped his elbows and knees with them—his reflexes had all gone back to normal. When I scratched the soles of his feet, his toes curled down—the normal response, no more Babinski sign. I lifted him from the table to the floor and asked him to hop on one leg, which he did easily. I bent down, reached around him, and gently put my hands on the back of his neck to see if it was still stiff. He initially pulled away, but with his dad's encouragement he cooperated. His neck was more flexible than before, but there was a hint of slight stiffness at the extremes of movement, and he winced a little. But he didn't cry this time.

I told him I was finished, and he scrambled back up onto the chair and began eating his pizza. I was mystified. Could the cyst have ruptured, removing the pressure on the spinal cord? I asked Enel if Davidson had fallen or had any other trauma.

He said he hadn't.

I asked if he had gotten any treatment, wondering if they'd sought out a traditional healer. I thought most traditional treatments in Haiti involved herbal remedies, but I wondered if maybe they had some ritual where they manipulated his neck in some way that had ruptured the cyst.

He said they hadn't done anything like that.

"M te priye anpil," Enel said matter-of-factly. ("I prayed a lot.")

I sat back down at the table across from them, lost in thought as they ate in silence. Anne and I had spent months trying to convince Mark (the neurosurgeon who offered to operate on Davidson) and the Boston Children's Hospital staff that we would come through with the passports. Now the patient we'd been advocating for didn't have anything wrong with him anymore! Anne and I had both had several staticky calls with Enel over the past few months to see how things were going with the passport situation. Why hadn't he ever mentioned that Davidson had gotten better?

My thoughts were spinning. I tried to think rationally. As a first step, we could repeat the CT scan. If the cyst had disappeared, perhaps Davidson had lucked out and the delayed passport was a blessing in disguise, saving him a risky surgery for a problem that would have resolved on its own. But what if the cyst was still there? I had to know.

Once they had finished their pizza, we set off through the open field that leads to the dirt road to the hospital. We passed the tree-branch soccer goalposts, some scrawny sleeping dogs, and a few bony mules and cows tethered to wooden posts, lazily swatting flies with their tails. I asked Enel what kind of work he did, and he told me he was a middle school science teacher. He had three other children aside from Davidson who all lived with him. I asked who would take care of them if he and Davidson came to Boston. He said their mother's sister would stay with them. He didn't mention their mother, and I didn't ask.

When Davidson's scan was finished, I brought him and Enel back to the staff house to rest and then jogged back to the hospital to wait for the images to be ready for review. If the cyst had somehow vanished, this would be miraculous and simplify the situation. But suppose it was still there—would Mark perform this delicate and risky operation if the scan was abnormal but the child appeared normal?

I imagined how I would react if I was meeting Davidson and Enel for the first time. Enel would recount the history of Davidson becoming quadriplegic over three years and then recovering spontaneously. He might bring a report from a CT scan revealing the cyst. Or maybe he wouldn't have been able to get a scan. I probably wouldn't even think about sending a normal-appearing child for surgery. "I have no explanation for what happened," I might say, "but I'm glad he's better and I'll keep following him." Another neurologic mystery, I would think. Haiti has plenty of them.

But today wasn't the first time I had met Davidson. I had seen him when he was severely disabled. And the clock was ticking on funds allotted for him to get neurosurgery for free. Would there be a bias to intervene, given all we'd been through—Enel for his passport and Davidson's, Mark and the Boston Children's administration for their efforts to make good on their soon-to-expire free-care budget for the year?

I thought about how I had imagined Janel to be a walking, talking college student only to discover just how bad off he was the moment before we brought him to the US for surgery. But Davidson's case seemed to be proceeding in the opposite direction—he had been fully paralyzed from the neck down when I met him, and now he was completely normal at the moment we were going to send him for surgery!

As I had progressed from medical school through residency to independent practice as a neurologist, I grew increasingly aware of how often things seemed ambiguous in medicine. Patients' cases were almost never straightforward, diagnoses were rarely definitive, treatment decisions were hardly ever clear-cut. In Haiti, practicing medicine felt even more perplexing, the patients more enigmatic, the clinical reasoning more baffling. There were no cases in the textbooks like Davidson's. And I had no idea what the right thing to do for him would be.

The CT scan showed that Davidson's cyst was still there. It looked exactly the same. I let Mark know that Davidson had miraculously recovered, but his scan showed that the cyst was unchanged. I asked him what he thought we should do. He replied:

> I don't know what the right answer is. I would say that, unequivocally, for a child that was here in the US we would operate for a large cyst that had caused such profound symptoms. My main concern is that his neurological decline, from which he thankfully recovered, will not be an isolated event, and that the next time, or the one after that, he might not recover. I do suspect that the care would be easy, with one surgery and not a lot of follow up, but the case is so unusual that this is hard to predict. It is definitely reasonable to wait and see what happens, but the trouble is a local Boston case could get right back in for emergent treatment if something happened, and we know this child cannot.

I felt reluctant to send a normal-appearing child for surgery. But I'm not a neurosurgeon, and so I couldn't trust my risk-averse anxiety, an anxiety made worse by all that had happened with Janel. If an expert pediatric neurosurgeon like Mark thought Davidson was at high risk for recurrence of his paralysis and the surgery was straightforward, I trusted his judgment.

I was headed back to Boston and thought it was best that the local pediatricians present the neurosurgeon's impression and recommendation for surgery to Enel, communicating the caveat of the no-right-answer scenario and that this might be a unique window of opportunity in which he could get the operation for free.

As I waited at the staff house for my ride to the airport, I got a text message from the HUM pediatricians that they had discussed all of this with Enel, and after thinking it over for a few days, he decided to go ahead with the surgery. They said our colleagues were working on expediting his passport.

"You know Dr. Michelle?" the driver asked me in English as we pulled out of the staff house onto the dirt road toward the route out of Mirebalais.

"Yes, she's one of my heroes!" I said. "She's the person who got me started working in Haiti."

"Yes!" he replied enthusiastically. "She has done so much for Haiti! Tell her I said hello when you see her in Boston."

"I sure will," I replied. I leaned my head back on the headrest and dozed off as we made our way to the airport.

"*Gade! Moun mouri!*" the driver said, pointing out the window of the PIH van. ("Look! A dead person!")

I opened my eyes to see what he was talking about. We had just made it to the straight highway into Port-au-Prince after whipping through the winding mountain roads from Mirebalais.

On the side of the road, a few feet from a motorcycle, there was a man in a red T-shirt and gray pants lying facedown. A small crowd of people had gathered around him.

"Motorcycle accident?" I asked the driver as we drove past. I presumed the unfortunate man had gotten thrown to the ground from the motorcycle that lay on its side nearby.

"No, it was a *krim!*" he said.

"Cream?" I asked.

"Yes, they killed him," he said.

"Ah, crime." I hadn't heard the word "crime" in Creole before—it's pronounced "cream"—and it took me a moment to register it. "But how do you know?" I asked.

"Didn't you see his hands were tied behind his back with a cord?"

I hadn't seen that. "But there are so many people around, and it's such a busy road . . ."

"That's why they put the body here. To scare people."

"But then wouldn't everyone have seen them do it?"

"No, they didn't kill him here." He laughed at my naïveté. "They just threw the body here overnight. There are no lights on the road so it would be very dark, and not many people are on this road at night."

"Oh . . ." I said, trailing off, disturbed. I watched the brightly colored *taptaps* streaming by, overflowing with people in the morning rush. I read the slogans written across the tops of their windshields as they passed: *Don de Dieu* (Gift of God), *Sang de Jesus* (Blood of Jesus), *Foi de Job* (Job's faith), *Humilité* (Humility) . . .

"They tied his hands behind his back and beat his head with a rock," he explained. "Maybe he was a robber. Or maybe he got into a fight with someone. There must be some story."

I stayed silent. I had seen people die in the hospital many times, but a dead body lying on the side of the road? That was a first for me.

"In your country, the police would come and investigate the scene, right?" he began. "Even by analyzing the cord they tied his hands with, or the rock they killed him with, they would find the person who killed him. But not here, no! They will just come and take the body to the morgue. No investigation! No nothing!" His voice had risen in pitch and volume, cracking at points. "There's no structure, no order! Mm! So people are running around like cannibals in the wild, killing each other with rocks! *Tèt chaje!*"

He continued with equal intensity. "You know why people act like that in this country? You know why? Because in one hundred people, you know how many can eat every day? Two or three!" He had stretched out the last three words slowly, and then he repeated them quickly at a higher pitch: "Two or three! And out of a thousand people in Haiti, do you know how many people have jobs? Again, two or three. Two or three! The rest? *Miser!*" ("Poverty"; literally "misery.") "If you don't have a job and you don't have any food, what choice do you have? You steal, you fight, maybe you even kill someone. People need to *work!*"

He fell silent as we weaved in and out of traffic: motorcycles, *taptaps*, dump trucks filled with large stones. We drove along a section of the road with open plains on both sides, a few banana trees in the distance, their leaves swaying gently.

"Look at this land," he said. *"Terre vierge!"* ("Virgin land!") "Why doesn't the government develop this land for the people? Give them some land! Give them some jobs! Why not?! You want to know why not? Because they only serve themselves! They put the money in their own pockets! These candidates, you know what they do? They distribute guns to the people to kill the supporters of their opponents. They pay poor people a thousand gourdes"—about twenty dollars—"to vote for them. But who pays the *politicians*? Who pays *them*?! The bourgeoisie. The bourgeoisie finance the campaigns of the senators, the presidents. And so who do they serve when they are elected? The bourgeoisie! And the rest of the people? *Miser!* They live in *miser*. Only two or three out of a hundred can eat! Only two or three out of a thousand have jobs! So many problems in this country!" He shook his head and made a clicking sound. "So many problems," he said again, his tone calming. "Big problems."

We arrived at the airport. The driver smiled, leaned toward me, and slapped his hand into mine in a firm handshake.

"Safe flight, and don't forget to say hi to Dr. Michelle for me in Boston!" he said.

"I'll do that," I replied as I got my suitcase out of the back seat.

I walked through the crowds in the airport lobby to the ticket counter in a daze, the driver's intense rant ringing in my ears, the image of the facedown corpse lingering in my mind's eye.

The agent entered my information into the computer and looked up at me. "Boston?" he asked with a Creole accent (*Beau-stone*).

"Boston," I confirmed.

Boarding pass in hand, I made my way to the security line. Everyone was talking, laughing, showing each other pictures on their phones. Did they know that outside, not far away, a murder victim had been tossed onto the side of the road?

Life is so much more fragile than people realize, I thought. Skin tears, bones break, organs fail, tumors invade. Doctors see that bodies can break down just like anything else in this world. So fragile. *"Li la!"* Janel's mom had said excitedly. ("He's here!") *Just barely*, I remembered thinking. *"Li mouri!"* the ladies had laughed when we ran over the chicken that tried to cross the road. ("It died!") Days later Francky had died before he could cross to the other side—*lòt bò a*—for treatment. The space between *"Li la"* and *"Li mouri"*—between here and not here—is connected by such a thin, thin thread. Like the thin, thin thread of spinal cord connecting Davidson's brain to his body. But somehow that thread seemed to be working. For now. *Li la*—he's here. Miraculously recovered. But how long would his luck last? It was impossible to know. This unfortunate boy had been completely paralyzed—wasn't surgery worth the risk if it could prevent that from happening again? But now he was completely normal—what if the surgery made him paralyzed again? After all that had happened with Janel, were we out of our minds to try to bring another patient to Boston for neurosurgery?

Life is so much more fragile than people realize, I thought again. *Especially here.*

A few days after I returned to Boston, Enel and Davidson arrived, and I went to visit them at the Ronald McDonald House. Enel was dressed in a black suit with a white button-down shirt, and Davidson was in a white suit and white button-down shirt. Both wore perfectly shined black dress shoes, and both had their hair closely cropped. I remembered that Janel had also arrived in Boston in his Sunday best. The last time I'd seen Davidson and Enel, we'd walked on dirt roads past emaciated farm animals in Mirebalais.

While Enel told me about their trip, Davidson ran in circles around his legs, occasionally stopping to peek at me from around his dad's thigh as he had done about a month prior in Mirebalais. He flashed an adorable ear-to-ear smile, revealing that he had lost his top two front teeth since I last saw him.

I smiled back at him, but then felt a twinge in my stomach. I thought back to the moment Janel had arrived in Boston and how I had knelt by his gurney in the emergency room, feeling overjoyed that we had managed to get him from one of the poorest parts of the world to a high-tech Harvard hospital. I never could have imagined in that moment how things would ultimately play out for him despite my best intentions. I tried to maintain my smile at Davidson but felt a sickening sense of uneasiness. We were about to send this adorable, completely normal boy for a major surgery at the junction of his brain and spinal cord.

On the day of surgery, Anne sat with Enel in the waiting room across the hall from the operating rooms during breaks in her workday, bringing him food. When I finished work in the late afternoon, I headed across the street to Boston Children's. By the time I arrived, Anne and

Enel were the only ones in the waiting room. They were sitting next to each other in silence. Anne said they hadn't heard any updates for a few hours. She went back to work, and I took her seat next to Enel, who was quietly looking at his phone.

"Can I get you something to eat or drink?" I asked.

"No," he replied softly, still looking at his phone. He seemed anxious, understandably.

We sat in silence.

"What are you reading?" I asked. He showed me his phone, on which a Bible app was open to Psalm 103 ("Bless the Lord, O my soul, and all that is within me, bless his holy name. Bless the Lord, O my soul, and forget not all his benefits"). He showed me how the app could be searched by chapter and verse. He went back to reading—praying, I presumed—and I decided to stop asking him questions. I took out my phone and caught up on email.

An hour passed. It had gotten dark outside the windows of the waiting room. We still hadn't heard anything. I checked with a staff member, who said the operation was finished, but they were still waiting for Davidson to wake up.

Finally, Mark came into the waiting room from the operating room. Despite countless emails back and forth, we had never met. He looked much younger than I had anticipated for a department chair—I estimated he was in his late forties. He smiled warmly beneath his circular thin-rimmed glasses as he entered.

"You must be Aaron," he said. "Nice to finally meet you."

I stood and shook hands with him. "Great to meet you in person," I said. "Thanks so much again."

Enel stood nervously, looking at Mark wide-eyed, his jaw tight, his face pulled taught over his high cheekbones. He shook Mark's hand timidly.

Mark pulled up a chair, and we all sat down, facing each other.

"I can translate," I offered.

"Great," Mark said. "Everything went well," he began calmly. I translated. Some of the tension began to leave Enel's face, but his eyes remained unblinkingly focused on Mark.

Mark turned to me, "The cyst was slightly adherent to the upper cervical spinal cord, but we were able to dissect it away. That's what took longer than expected."

He spoke as calmly and casually as if he was describing putting up wallpaper or changing a flat tire. But he had just carved a cyst off the region at the intersection between the brain and the rest of the body. Any missteps could have paralyzed Davidson from the neck down.

"What do you think it is?" I asked him.

"I don't know, but it deflated pretty easily," he replied. "It didn't look like a tumor. We sent it to pathology, so we'll find out soon."

Mark turned back to Enel. "He's still waking up, but he's moving everything just fine," he said. "You can see him when he gets upstairs in an hour or so."

I translated. Enel nodded, the fright in his large eyes beginning to fade, leaving fatigue in its wake.

I admired Mark's style. He appeared unrushed despite it being well into the evening, and despite having spent most of his day operating within the space of a few inches.

"Do you have any questions for Dr. Proctor?" I asked Enel.

He shook his head slowly. Then he looked at me and said, *"Di li mesi anpil e Bondye ap beni li."*

"He says to tell you thank you very much and may God bless you," I said to Mark.

Mark smiled and stood, shaking hands with Enel and then with me.

"Thank you so much for taking care of him," I said. "I'm so sorry again for all of the challenges getting him here."

"Not at all," he said, smiling warmly. "Thank you for all you and Anne did to make it happen."

Enel and I collected his belongings and rode the elevator up to the

ICU to wait for Davidson. When he arrived, he was sleeping soundly. He'd been under anesthesia the whole day, so that was expected. Enel was able to stay with him on a foldout cot in the room. It was getting late, and I told Enel I would come back to see them in the morning before work.

The next morning, I found Enel leaning over the bed of the brightly lit white hospital room. Davidson was sobbing the Haitian cry of pain—"*OO-eeeeee . . . AY-eeeee . . .*"—a wrenching wail I knew all too well from the emergency room at HUM. He seemed to be moving both arms and legs, and I breathed a sigh of relief. But Enel looked as distraught as he had appeared the day before when we were waiting for the surgery to end.

Enel said Davidson was in a lot of pain, but the nurses were giving him medicine for it. With even the smallest movements, Davidson would scream in agony. "'Son-son, 'Son-son," Enel kept saying, trying to soothe him between his cries. He gently turned Davidson onto his side, revealing a large gauze bandage running from the back of his head to the base of his neck.

"This is normal after such a big surgery," I tried to reassure Enel. He didn't look reassured.

Davidson's nurse came in and said she was going to give him pain medication through his IV. I translated for Enel, who nodded. I had to run to work but told Enel I'd visit again. As I walked down the hallway out of the ICU, I heard Davidson's cries fade to whimpering as the medication took effect and Enel continued to comfort him: "Okay, 'Son-son. Okay, 'Son-son."

When I went back to visit them the next day, Davidson's nurse told me he had been transferred out of the ICU to the ward overnight, a good sign. I found Davidson in his new room, sitting up in bed. Enel was feeding him from a hearty hospital meal tray. Davidson watched cartoons with rapt attention while he ate.

"*Li mye!*" I said, smiling as I entered. ("He's better!")

"*Wi li mye*," Enel agreed, looking exhausted but much more relaxed than the prior day. ("Yes, he's better.")

"Can I get you some lunch?" I offered.

"Dr. Anne gave me these," he said, taking some meal tickets for the Boston Children's cafeteria out of his shirt pocket.

"Oh, great," I said, amazed at how Anne always thought of everything. "So you've been to the cafeteria?"

"No, I haven't gone yet," he said.

"You haven't gone to the cafeteria in two days?" I asked, concerned.

"No, because then who would be here with Davidson?" he asked matter-of-factly.

"It's okay. You can go," I said. "His nurse is here."

"But she's not here all of the time," he said.

"So you haven't eaten in two days?" I asked.

He looked at me sheepishly and shrugged.

In Haiti, as in many poor countries with limited hospital staff, family members are expected to provide much of the bedside monitoring and care when a patient is hospitalized. We hadn't thought to explain to Enel that the nurses were keeping a constant eye on Davidson, so he didn't have to stay at his son's bedside around the clock.

"It's not like Haiti," I assured him. "The nurses will take care of everything. You are allowed to leave him if you need to."

He looked at me skeptically or confused—I couldn't tell. I went to find Davidson's nurse and explained that Enel hadn't left his son's bedside in days because he was afraid to leave him alone. I asked if she could stay with Davidson for a few minutes so we could go down to the cafeteria. She agreed, and Enel and I went off to find him something to eat.

As we rode the elevator down, I thought about just how far away from home Enel was. He had such extraordinary courage to get on a plane and go to a place where he knew nobody, for a high-risk surgery on his perfectly normal son, advised by a surgeon he had never met, communicated to him by a person he had spoken with only briefly.

Enel had placed unbelievable trust in me, in us, in the system. Not having children myself, I could only imagine the depths of fear and anxiety that must come from seeing one's own child suffer. Still, I wondered how I would react if a visiting foreigner I'd met for just a few minutes told me, "Just come to my country, we'll take care of your child for free—medical care, flights, food, housing, no problem. Just come. We'll be waiting for you at the airport." Looking at Enel as he watched the elevator numbers descend to the lobby, I was filled with admiration for him. Such incredible bravery and faith to be willing to take a chance to help his child. Such love and devotion to forgo eating for a few days to make sure his son would not be left alone and afraid.

The elevator doors opened, and I showed Enel the landmarks on the way to the cafeteria so he could return there on his own. We used his meal tickets from Anne to get him food for the next few meals and then rode the elevator back up to Davidson's room. His nurse was feeding him his lunch while he continued to be mesmerized by the cartoons on television. I thanked the nurse, said goodbye to Enel and Davidson, and headed back to work.

Davidson was discharged, pain-free, within a few days. He walked out of the hospital just as he had walked in. Mark felt that it would be best to keep him in the US for a month or so, since it would be hard to get him back to Boston from Haiti if something unexpected happened. Anne had discovered from talking with Enel that his wife—Davidson's mom—was living in Florida, so we offered to send Enel and Davidson there for the month, which they were very excited about. After that month, we would bring them back to Boston for a follow-up visit. By then we would have the pathology results that we hoped would confirm Mark's impression in the operating room, that the cyst was benign and no further treatment would be needed. If all was okay, we planned to send them back to Haiti at that time. It looked like this was going to be much more straightforward than Janel's care had been, passport drama notwithstanding.

I slipped back into my normal life, the one that didn't involve run-

ning back and forth to Boston Children's or the Ronald McDonald
House before work, between patients, or after work.

A week later, I received an email from Mark:

> Fascinating turn of events on Davidson. The pathology is a
> neurenteric cyst, which I've never seen present like this, both
> in the cervical region, and dorsal to the spinal cord. It means
> that surgery was absolutely the right thing—this was going to
> grow and paralyze him without surgery. Thanks.

I'd never heard of a neurenteric cyst. "Enteric" generally refers to
the gastrointestinal system, but I thought it must have some different
meaning here. When I looked it up, I discovered that a neurenteric cyst
was indeed gut tissue that ended up in the wrong place during embry-
ological development. They are rare: about one percent of spinal cord
tumors, which themselves are very rare. Normally when these residual
gastrointestinal cysts occur in the spine they arise in the thoracic region (at the level of the gut) and in front of the spinal cord (where the
gut is), not at the top of the spinal cord and behind it (where Davidson's
was). A rare entity in a doubly rare location.

Fortunately, the cyst was benign. Davidson wouldn't need any
chemotherapy, radiation, or further surgeries—he was cured.

Enel and Davidson came back from Florida a month later and spent
one last night at the Ronald McDonald House before their final appointment with Mark. I went to visit them and found them in the living
room. Enel was relaxing on a couch, watching a football game with
a distant cousin who Enel's wife had told him was living in Boston.
Davidson was running around the living room, diving onto the couch
and rolling around on it, then running around again, giggling each
time he bounced on the couch's cushions. It was only when he stopped
long enough to look at the television that I could see the well-healed
scar running down the back of his neck. I thought about how the plan
to get Davidson to Boston for surgery had nearly fallen apart several

times with all the twists and turns—the paralysis that mysteriously resolved, the lost passport, the near miss on losing his chance for free care. As he raced around the room so fast that he became a blur of arms, legs, and a blue T-shirt, I smiled and shook my head, relieved that somehow it had all worked out.

A few days later, father and son returned to Haiti, just over a month after they had arrived in Boston.

Shortly after they got home, I received a text message from Enel. He told me Davidson was doing well and was back in school and playing sports. He concluded:

> *Se Bondye map di merci avan, epi apre, se tout dokte ke Bondye te fe ede mwen, paske mwen tap priye anpil pou chirirgie a te posib.* (It is God who I thank first, and then after, all the doctors who God made help me, because I prayed so much for the surgery to be possible.)

As touched as I was by his message, I felt we couldn't really take credit for curing Davidson's paralysis since he had mysteriously recovered before the operation. But he had made it through the process unscathed, and now he and his father could live a life free from fear that he could one day become paralyzed again. After Janel's disappointing outcome and Francky's death, it looked like Davidson was going to be our first success story, our first big save.

15

Working with the HUM rehab team, Janel got to the point where he could take a few steps with assistance. But he didn't progress to nearly the level he had reached after his previous course of rehabilitation a few months earlier. The rehab team felt he had plateaued, and they needed to make his bed available for another patient. They wanted to continue his physical therapy through home visits, but Janel's mother lived too far away. Eager to continue with the therapy, his mother found a spare room in a house in Mirebalais that was owned by a friend of Janel's father, and she moved there with Janel.

When the physical therapist arrived to work with Janel the following week, he was shocked by Janel's living conditions. The physical therapist told one of the HUM social workers to evaluate the situation right away.

The social worker found Janel and his mother in a one-room shack made of overlapping palisaded sheet-metal panels, rusted and ragged. The doorless entrance faced onto a small dirt footpath. The social worker's steps leading up to the shack kicked up a cloud of dust that hung in the doorway.

Inside, the social worker found Janel lying on a mattress on a dirt floor. His mother had put some plastic bags under the mattress to try to keep it from getting wet when the rain turned the floor from dirt to mud. Janel looked like he had lost weight. His mother told the social worker that she was in debt to many of her new neighbors from asking to borrow food for Janel. In spite of this, she was still not able to feed him every day. Janel's father hadn't visited in over two weeks, and the owner of the house said he needed the room back because his children would be visiting him soon. Janel's mother didn't know where they would live after this. She said Janel was starting to walk and talk a little, but he still needed complete support to get around.

Concluding a report on his home visit, the social worker wrote:

The situation is both serious and urgent. This is a patient who needs a lot of support because of his level of disability. His mother is aged and ravaged by miserable poverty, she's not well nourished, she's not well housed, she's not certain what tomorrow will bring. That's the reality of Janel's life. That's why this is an emergency. So we need a plan. I remain available to help in any way with my team so Janel can have a better life.

The report included a list of both short-term needs (renting an adequate shelter, financial assistance for food, and some basic furniture and utensils) and long-term goals (finding or building Janel and his mother an accessible house in an accessible location and trying to find some type of employment for Janel's mother).

When I discussed the report with Père Eddy, the priest and psychologist who directs the HUM mental health team, he lamented, "Have we managed to cure this boy's tumor with surgery, radiation, and chemotherapy in the US only to have him die of hunger back home in Haiti?!"

It was a tragic truth. After all of the complex and costly medical and logistical coordination, we were failing at the most simple and inexpensive of interventions: housing and food.

I remembered back when I had envisioned Janel as a mildly affected college student, a straightforward big save, a chance to apply the PIH principles I aspired to. But every turn had a twist, each decision was overshadowed by a dilemma, and it was unclear if we had even really helped him in any significant way. Though Davidson's success story had given me hope for how much modern medical care can change a patient's life, Janel's case was a painful reminder that medicine is powerless when it narrowly focuses on treating a disease, neglecting to address the patient's social and economic circumstances.

"They always say in development work that you have to teach people to fish, not just give them a fish, or else it isn't sustainable," Père Eddy continued. "But do you know what, dear Aaron? Sometimes you just have to give them a fish! We can't wait for it to be sustainable. In the meantime, they must eat!"

Fortunately, PIH runs Program on Social and Economic Rights (POSER), which serves both purposes: giving out fish and teaching people to fish. One of the core tenets of PIH's model of care delivery is considering health beyond the limited notion of disease. Patients are more likely to get sick and less likely to receive healthcare if they are poor. So helping poor patients recover from disease and prevent future illness requires supporting them socioeconomically: housing, food, clean water, sanitation, employment, education, clothes. POSER would be lifesaving for Janel and his mother, but such socioeconomic interventions are complicated. In PIH's description of POSER, they state:

> Jealousy among people who do not receive a house or housing support through the program is another common challenge. . . . POSER staff should inform the community about why certain people have been selected to receive a house, while not violating the privacy or confidentiality regarding the medical condition of the recipient, if applicable. Being an advocate for POSER beneficiaries, and minimizing any conflicts that POSER activities may provoke is part of the job of POSER staff.

If we had a new home constructed for Janel and his mother and provided them with an allowance, would others in their community wonder why they had gotten special treatment while everyone else remained hungry in decrepit shacks? Would we be putting Janel and his mother at risk for mistreatment or robbery by intervening in this way?

When policymakers speak of compromises that must be made due to limited resources, Paul Farmer is known to counter that we are in fact in a time when there are more resources available than at any other time in history, but they just aren't equitably distributed: the compromises and limited resources are for the poor, while everyone else enjoys the excess. Part of Paul Farmer's message, as I'd always understood it, is not to forget the individual patients who make up the statistics of public health and policy. And yet in trying to reduce the suffering of one single individual, to right one inequitable wrong, what unintended consequences might lurk beyond? If we can't resolve inequity for everyone at once, do our actions to help individuals create ripple effects that only serve to create new inequities?

Through POSER, PIH allotted funds to build or rent a new house in Mirebalais for Janel and his mother and provide them with a living stipend. But the process of performing a needs assessment and psychosocial evaluation, using this information to determine how best to help them, finding an appropriate location for them to live, and negotiating with the local community would take time. And it wasn't just logistics that made the process slow. When I checked in with the HUM mental health team about their progress, a colleague wrote back apologizing for the delay. The bus their team used to travel between PIH/ZL sites had been attacked at gunpoint along its usual route. Nobody had been hurt, but after terrorizing the staff, the attackers had broken the bus's windows and set it on fire. The psychologist who wrote to me about this event concluded her email:

It was Scary!

People are traumatized!

It is a Shame for the image of our Country!

We have enough problems—we did not need those things.
The worst is that we can't even guarantee It won't happen
again and again.

Sorry!

It was going to be a while before we'd have a safe situation for Janel
and his mother.

Père Eddy moved things along nonetheless. He wrote to us:

> We need to move from words to actions. The list of needs is
> long, but we don't have to do everything at once. Let's start
> with the basic need of food support.

He and Michelle secured funding from HUM for an allowance of
five thousand Haitian gourdes (about seventy-eight dollars) per month
for Janel and his mother. Père Eddy wrote to me:

> A small victory, a first step. But the fight for Janel's life must
> continue!

Seventy-eight dollars per month seemed like an insultingly low sum
to me. Could they really survive on this? But after one of the HUM
social workers delivered the first payment to them, he wrote to us:

> This manna arrived just in time. The joy expressed by Janel's
> mother cannot be described in words. However, the larger
> problems are not yet taken care of. We must continue in our
> efforts to bring better conditions to this patient's life.

Just over $2.50 per day was next to nothing. But compared to zero, it was an infinite improvement for Janel and his mother.

———————

"W se Doktè Aaron?" asked a young man as I was leaving HUM for the day. ("Are you Dr. Aaron?")

I didn't recognize him. He looked like he was in his early thirties and was well dressed in a loose, checkered button-down shirt that was untucked and hung over pressed dark jeans. The first few buttons of his shirt were left open, revealing a gold chain. He had thin-rimmed glasses, and his hair was shaved to the scalp, giving his head a reflective shine in the midday sun. Did I know him? I wasn't sure.

He introduced himself as Ricardo and said he was working with the HUM mental health team on Janel's case. I recognized his name from emails, but I hadn't met him before. He was the person who had found Janel's new house, negotiated a good price with the landlord, and brought Janel and his mom their monthly stipend.

I shook his hand and thanked him for all he had done for Janel. He said he was going to do a needs assessment for Janel and his mother and follow up with me by email about what still had to be purchased for their new home. He asked if I could help him move it forward, and I assured him I would.

After I returned to Boston, I received an email from Ricardo that included a long list of the items he recommended purchasing and their prices. I thanked him and forwarded the list to Père Eddy and his team. Père Eddy replied moments later:

> Pay close attention! In the needs assessment for Janel, we should be very professional. I looked at this list of things we need, and I'm not certain some of these are priorities! Between being able to not go hungry in the long term and having satellite TV, which is more important? If we fulfilled all

of the demands on this list, what money would we have left for Janel and his family's true needs?

I was shocked. I looked over the list more carefully. Nestled among items such as curtains, chairs, a refrigerator, and a fan were two separate line items for televisions: one satellite, one regular.

I apologized to Père Eddy that I hadn't looked at the list in detail before forwarding it. We received increasingly frustrated and angry emails from Ricardo about not getting the necessary funds to buy the items he had asked for in Janel's needs assessment.

I was perplexed and asked Martineau about the situation the next time I was back in Haiti. "Why did Ricardo think Janel needed a satellite TV?"

"Of course he doesn't need a satellite TV," Martineau said and laughed. "Ricardo was planning to steal the extra money." He looked at me incredulously as if this should have been obvious and I was naïve for not having figured it out.

"Wow . . ." I replied, shocked.

"He's not all bad," Martineau said. "He did a good job finding the house for Janel and his mother, and he worked hard to negotiate a good price in the community since he is from the region. But then he was stealing a little bit of their stipend each month. Janel's mother told me, so we did not allow him to deliver it anymore. Then he tried to steal from us again by sending this list with the two TVs."

"If everyone knows he's trying to steal, why do you still work with him?" I asked.

Martineau smiled. "You see, a long time ago, he was very sick. A very severe case. He was Dr. Paul Farmer's patient. Dr. Paul saved him and wanted to give him some work, so we cannot fire him. You know Dr. Paul. If we say, 'But he is stealing from us,' he will reply, 'It's not his fault, it is poverty that makes him do that, so you have to fix the poverty.'" He laughed. "You can't win the debate with him!"

"I can imagine." I laughed too. I had found myself in a debate with Paul Farmer just a few days before.

"Paul Farmer is here! Paul Farmer is here!"

I looked up from my laptop to see a young American woman standing in the doorway, a medical student who was living in Haiti for the year, working for PIH. It was a Saturday morning, and I was catching up on email with my feet up in the only air-conditioned conference room at HUM. The room is occupied all day each weekday for important administrative meetings, but during the weekend it's an ideal place to work—quiet, empty, cool, good Wi-Fi signal.

"He's here right now?" I asked, looking down at my Haiti weekend clothes: a ratty white undershirt, faded blue cargo pants, and a beat-up old pair of mud-crusted tennis shoes. "I'm, um, a bit underdressed for the occasion," I said and chuckled.

"Whatever," she replied and laughed. "He's visiting with some donors. You gotta come! He wants everyone working here to be there!" She ran off.

I had met Paul Farmer a few times after lectures he had given, but we'd never had a conversation. I was just one of the many groupies who would line up to shake his hand. In the field of global health, it was like meeting a rock star. He always looked each person in the eye when he shook hands with them and repeated the person's name after they introduced themselves ("Nice to meet you, Aaron"). It must have been his way of registering the name and face in photographic memory, because the second time I shook hands with him in his receiving line of admiring fans after a lecture, he said, "Thank you for the work you do, Aaron." I wondered if he really knew what I was doing or if it was just a stock phrase he had for the many young members of his fan club. Either way, I had been impressed that he remembered my name, since the first post-lecture handshake had been over a year earlier.

I walked out of the conference room into the stuffy late-morning heat of the administrative area at HUM. Sure enough, there he was. In his late fifties, Paul has closely cropped graying hair that forms a receding widow's peak. Seeing him up close, I was struck by the sharp angle of his nose, on which small rimless glasses were perched. His face looked slightly red, as if he had just shaved or was slightly sunburned, or both. He was dressed casually in a tan safari shirt buttoned to the top. My pulse quickened as I approached this living legend.

Paul was sitting across from two American doctors who were visiting to facilitate a training program in the HUM emergency room. I quietly pulled up a chair to the side of the three of them. The doctors Paul was speaking with were raising concerns about the lack of access to certain lab tests they felt were needed for patient care at HUM. Paul responded by explaining how a new lab they were building at HUM was going to address those concerns and beyond.

"The new lab is going to revolutionize diagnostic capacity in Haiti," Paul said. "Just like having the first publicly available CT scanner in Haiti here at HUM has done." Then he turned quickly toward where I was sitting and pointed his index finger at me. "Especially true for a neurologist. Am I right, Aaron?"

I blushed, startled to hear my name, surprised and flattered that he knew it, let alone that he knew I was a neurologist. I wondered if he really remembered or whether he had been briefed on who was at HUM at the time and what they were doing. However he knew me, I suddenly realized that if there was ever a moment to bring up our challenges trying to get neurosurgical patients to Boston, this was it. I had started advocating for the three brain tumor patients I'd met on a prior trip, but the process was slow going, and I thought help from Paul's position of influence could make a huge difference.

"The CT has definitely been a game changer for neurology here," I began, "but it has also raised some ethical dilemmas."

"Which ethics—*whose* ethics—are you referring to?" Paul quipped with a half smile, cocking his head slightly to one side with jerky, birdlike rapidity.

I kicked myself for using the word "ethical," remembering that an entire section of a 680-page anthology of Paul Farmer's essays has the phrase "A Critique of Medical Ethics" in its title. I certainly wasn't looking for a philosophical debate with one of the world's leading medical anthropologists. The reference list alone to the collection of his essays is 60 pages, longer than any essay I'd ever written. And it was Paul Farmer's work that had inspired me to be where I was at that very moment: working for PIH in Haiti. I didn't want to look stupid or offend him. I sidestepped his question and tried again.

"Well, in neurology, the CT . . ." I began haltingly. "I mean it's been amazing to have that resource, but . . . well . . . it's allowing us to diagnose things that we can't treat here, like—"

"Don't let anyone say you can't do something here," he interrupted with a slightly scolding tone. He seemed to be having fun sparring with me, but I was feeling flustered.

His replies were so rapid that I found it difficult to keep pace, so I tried to get my whole concern out in one breath. "The CT has allowed us to diagnose patients with really complex brain tumors that look like they could be big saves if we got them to surgery in the US, but the surgeries are just too risky to do here, and it's really challenging to get these patients to the US."

"Ah, you think history began when you arrived?" Paul asked playfully and chuckled. "We've been dealing with these issues for the last thirty years!" He took his cell phone out of his pants pocket. "I am going to send you something," he said. He fiddled briefly with his phone and then looked up from it with another birdlike jerk of his head, his blue eyes peering over his small circular spectacles. "Email address?" he asked.

I recited it and he typed it in. "Boom, sent!" he said giddily and put his phone away. "I just sent you the graduation speech I gave at USC last week."

"Great, thanks!" I said with a mix of genuine enthusiasm (an email from Paul Farmer!) and irritated frustration (what did this have to do with our conversation?).

"The speech is about how we separated conjoined twins here at HUM," he began. "Everyone said it couldn't be done here. *Shouldn't* be done here. Guess what? It's done! We did it! Here! Read the speech."

I could finally see where he was going with his argument. He thought we should be doing brain surgery at HUM. Paul wasn't the first person to suggest to me that we send neurosurgeons to Haiti instead of struggling to bring patients to the US, since the latter was much more logistically challenging, time-consuming, and costly. Luckily, I had needed to counter this argument before, so I had a well-worn response to why I didn't think this was a good idea.

"The surgery itself could technically be done here, but—" I began.

"In our beautiful modern operating rooms!" he interrupted exuberantly.

"But I'm afraid the patients would die postoperatively," I continued. "What if they develop diabetes insipidus? How could we monitor and react to that?" Diabetes insipidus—distinct from diabetes mellitus (which is what most people refer to when they say "diabetes")—is a condition in which miscommunication between the brain and kidneys causes the kidneys to spill massive amounts of sodium into the urine. It can occur after neurosurgery, requiring monitoring of blood and urine sodium levels as often as hourly to avoid fatal complications of fluid and electrolyte imbalances. There was no way to obtain labs and react to them that frequently at HUM. "I just think it would be safest for them to have surgery in the US," I concluded, hoping I'd made my case.

Paul made a half smile, half grimace as I spoke. Then he smiled fully. "That's what the new lab is for!" he said, pivoting back to the two emergency room doctors. "Like I was just telling my new friends here. Right guys?" He stood up. "Let's have lunch!"

I stood up too. Lunch would mean a larger crowd, and I saw my chance to try to get his help on this slipping away. Suddenly I thought of a way of framing my argument that might just convince him.

"But, Paul," I said, now standing just in front of him and looking up at him. "Don't you think the *preferential option for the poor* when it comes to these patients is to have their surgeries done in the US where we know it will be safest and lowest risk?"

His eyes darted quickly to the right for a split second and he blinked. *I got him*, I thought. How could he argue against one of his own core principles, the very words highlighted in the opening line of PIH's mission statement?

His eyes returned to mine. "Keep working on both fronts, then," he said soberly. "Keep trying on both fronts." He held my gaze with his for a brief moment longer. Then he nodded once and turned away to walk down the hall.

"*Nou grangou. Kikote manje a?*" he called out playfully. ("We're hungry. Where's the food?") The hospital staff preparing the food erupted in laughter. Paul had phrased it like the question of a hungry kid coming home from school.

I sat among a group of about a dozen local and expat staff, a few donors, and some of Paul's local friends around the conference room table where I'd had my feet up moments earlier. It had been converted into a dining table by the addition of a white tablecloth, place settings, and a buffet of rice and beans, goat stew, and *pikliz* (pickled cabbage, carrots, and peppers).

We listened to Paul with rapt attention as he held court on various topics. He talked about the new book he was working on, a critique of the global response to Ebola. "Umbrage will be taken," he said as he passed around the manuscript, a huge stack of pages with double-spaced type covered in notes scrawled in red ink. "Umbrage will be taken," he repeated.

He spoke of his three top goals for PIH in the coming year: completing the construction of the HUM clinical laboratory, building a new hospital in Liberia, and developing botanical gardens for the HUM grounds. The last one caught us all off guard, and he seemed to relish that. He paused for effect with a wry smile as we all looked at him, squinting, brows furrowed, confused at how creating a garden could be placed on the same level as the rebuilding of a health system in post-Ebola West Africa.

"I want HUM to be beautiful, not just functional," he finally said. "Don't our patients deserve that?"

I felt so privileged to be there, listening to the thoughts of this visionary hero who inspired a generation of health profession students—myself included—to pursue the goal of global health equity, to accompany the poor, to advocate for the marginalized. I caught myself smiling, remembering how blown away I had been when I read *Mountains Beyond Mountains*, the popular biography of Paul Farmer and his work with PIH. I couldn't believe I was sitting across the table from one of my idols. Then I recalled our debate before lunch. Why had he responded so disappointingly to my advocacy for some of our patients in Haiti to get surgery in the US? It just didn't make sense to me based on what I understood as his—and PIH's—principles.

That night, I brought my phone under my mosquito net to read the graduation speech that Paul had sent me earlier in the day. I recognized the jokey, punchy style from speeches I'd heard him give. He mixed tragic tales of doctors dying of Ebola in West Africa with a comical story of when he returned to the US from West Africa during the Ebola epidemic, causing chaos at the airport when the crew and passengers realized where he'd traveled from: "They didn't get Ebola, but they did miss their connections."

Finally, I located the paragraph that I thought was why he had wanted me to read the speech. He discussed the debate over whether the Haitian conjoined twins should be surgically separated in Haiti or in the US:

Ah, dear doctors of 2016! Debates ensued. You will see this often in your training and practice, especially when bold or audacious

*plans are proposed. But not everyone agreed with me . . . that this
course of action [doing the surgery in Haiti] was prudent or even
possible . . . I'd asked [a US-based] surgeon if this procedure could be
done in Haiti, since that's the point of building a university hospital
in the middle of the countryside: to provide care while training and
learning. That transferring the babies to Los Angeles or Boston
would have cost millions wasn't the main point, although finding
such resources, and visas and the like, would have been difficult. The
primary point was the babies' well-being. But it's worth noting that
the Haitian nurses and doctors who'd cared for [the mother] and her
babies wanted to see things through. And that could only happen in
Haiti. And it's not like the United States is a medical paradise or our
ICUs are free of highly drug-resistant pathogens. Research reported
just last month ranked medical error as the third-largest cause of
premature death. Right here in the US of A . . .*

He continued to describe the surgery itself at HUM in rousing
superlatives like "in beautiful surgical suites that were only a dream
when that country's hospitals came tumbling down only five years
previously" and "it looked like a typical first-world teaching hospital"
and "the girls' parents watched Haitian and American and Haitian-
American nurses and doctors and OR [operating room] techs make
medical history."

It was true that the successful separation of conjoined twins in Haiti
was extraordinary, but it had required an eighteen-person visiting surgical team working with a dozen local providers. And it was, well, not
brain surgery—the twins were connected at the liver. It was an amazing accomplishment, but attempting complex brain tumor surgery at
HUM seemed to me to be on another level.

I understood that Paul's career had been defined in part by proving
that what others thought was impossible was indeed possible. But he
had also taught us to think about how we could deliver the best care to
each and every patient in the world. He argued against the notion that

public health policies should prioritize cost-effective superficial solutions for whole populations, advocating instead for investment in systems to provide complete care for the individuals who make up those populations. Was he really suggesting we do neurosurgery at HUM to push the envelope, to prove it could be done in rural Haiti, even if patients could be at risk of dying in the process?

Paul Farmer is one of the world's leading experts in healthcare delivery in the poorest settings, with decades of experience all over the globe. At that point, I had been to Haiti just a handful of times over the preceding three years. Who was I to challenge him? If something didn't feel right to me, then clearly I must have been missing something.

A few months later, back working on the wards at Brigham, I ran into a doctor who had worked in Haiti since the early days of PIH. She asked me how things were going with my work there. I ended up venting my concerns to her about how we thought we were seeing neurologic complications of Zika virus infection in Haiti, but we weren't able to track the epidemic there because we couldn't seem to get patients' blood samples properly tested for Zika. I had worked myself up into a bit of a rant about how challenging and frustrating the situation was. I noticed she was smiling. She almost looked like she was about to laugh.

"I'm sorry," she said, trying to stifle her smile. "Go on."

"Oh, sorry, did I say something funny?" I asked, confused by her reaction.

"No, no. It's just that I can't believe I'm talking to a neurologist who works in Haiti," she said, "a neurologist who is complaining because we don't have the ability to rapidly diagnose an emerging infection!"

I didn't get it and looked at her quizzically.

"Can you imagine us there thirty years ago seeing patients under a tree?" she asked. "We had nothing. No specialists, no labs. Nothing! And now we have a neurologist! A neurologist who simply takes for granted that we have all the basics but doesn't think it's enough and wants to push to make it even better for our patients. It's wonderful!"

To her, the details I was able to be frustrated by were a reflection of just how far PIH's work in Haiti had come over the last three decades. This sudden expansion of perspective allowed me to finally make sense of my conversation with Paul Farmer at HUM a few months earlier.

Look around you, I imagined Paul had been trying to say to me. *It was "impossible" to provide HIV care in rural Haiti, but PIH did it. It was "impossible" to treat multidrug-resistant tuberculosis in the urban slums of Peru, but PIH did that too. And it was certainly "'impossible" to build a solar-powered three-hundred-bed hospital in rural Haiti, have it open and running at full capacity less than three years from the time the idea was first proposed, and—let's not forget—successfully separate conjoined twins there! But here we are. If you believe it's impossible, then it will be. Or you can choose to believe it's possible. Then you work on making it possible. The only failures are failures of imagination.*

In spite of this inspiring interpretation of what I thought Paul's message for me may have been during our debate, I still didn't think complex brain tumor surgery could be done safely at HUM. And the three patients we were advocating for didn't need surgery as urgently as Francky had, so we had time to keep trying to get them to Boston. I was determined to keep working on it to avoid a failure of imagination on that front.

We had to do better than we had done for Janel.

16

"Will you be able to recognize him?" Anne asked as we scanned the crowds of passengers streaming through the exit from customs at Logan Airport in Boston.

"Oh, I'll recognize him," I said, laughing. "I have seen Pasteur almost every time I've been to Haiti for the last two years!"

Pasteur Jean-Rémy—a forty-year-old pastor whom everyone just calls Pasteur—was one of the three patients for whom we'd been trying to arrange free care in Boston. He had a large tumor of his pituitary gland that was compressing the nerves to his eyes, resulting in blindness in his right eye and loss of peripheral vision in his left eye. We weren't sure if surgery would restore the vision he had lost, but we hoped it could save his remaining sliver of sight.

Given how complex and long—not to mention expensive—Janel's treatment had been, I had felt we needed to wait until Janel had returned home to approach the Brigham administration about more patients from Haiti. When we did begin advocating for them, things didn't seem to move as smoothly or as quickly as when we had proposed Janel's case.

Ian—the neurosurgeon who had operated on Janel—was eager to offer surgery for the three new patients. He thought their operations would all be far more straightforward than Janel's. I had seen all three patients and knew they were able to walk and care for themselves and had normal cognition, a very different starting point than with Janel. And yet somehow each step in the administrative process in Boston took longer. My suspicion was that these cases were going through a more rigorous vetting process because of all the challenges involved in Janel's care, though nobody ever said this. If that was the case, it was certainly understandable. I hadn't adequately anticipated the scope of Janel's care—not even close—and likely hadn't inspired confidence that I actually knew what I was doing as I scrambled to address challenges as they came up. And of course, every aspect of Janel's case had turned out very differently from the straightforward big save I had promised.

When Ian and I eventually received some initial encouraging signs from the hospital administration, I asked Martineau to reach out to the three patients to see who had passports. He was able to reach two of them: Pasteur and Nadège, the young woman with a tumor in her eye socket. Both had passports, both had worsening headaches, and both were eager to get treated. But Martineau couldn't reach the third patient, Jesula, the fifty-three-year-old woman with a large but benign tumor pressing on the top of her brain.

A few days later, he wrote to me that she had passed away.

I was infuriated that the slow administrative process had led to a patient with a benign, operable tumor dying so young. Another stupid death. Trying to convert anger to action, I informed the administration that they no longer needed to evaluate her for possible free care because she had died, and I asked for updates on the status of the other two patients' cases. I hoped to catalyze the process with this not-so-gentle reminder that these were not merely cases or cost estimates or risk assessments but actual human lives. I received an apology and assurance that the other two patients' files were being actively evaluated.

While all of this played out, Pasteur came to HUM nearly every time I was in Haiti, making the three-hour trip from the port town of Gonaïves to Mirebalais by *taptap*. When I had first met him, I explained that I would try to advocate on his behalf to get him surgery for free in the US, but I couldn't promise anything. Each time he came back, he told me he kept praying to God for help, and he knew his prayers would ultimately be answered. I wasn't so sure. I told him I was trying to help him, but it was a slow process and it wasn't up to me.

"*Apre Bondye se doktè!*" Pasteur would exclaim in response with a preacher's emphatic declamation. ("After God is the doctor!")

I had serious concerns that I wasn't going to live up to his expectations.

Once, when François—our first neurology trainee in Haiti—saw Pasteur's chart in the stack of the day's consults given to us by one of the HUM clinic nurses, he moved it to the bottom of the pile.

"Why did you do that?" I asked him.

"Because he always takes such a long time and then we fall so far behind!" he replied, slightly irritated. Then he looked away, shook his head, and added somberly, "And because it's just too depressing to see this poor pastor and not be able to do anything for him."

I felt ashamed too each time I saw Pasteur. Had I given him false hope in a situation in which I was not the ultimate decision-maker? Had I relied too heavily on our hospital as the only possible solution when I should have tried more broadly with other hospitals? But in a different hospital it would be harder for Michelle, Anne, and me to interface with the care team and advocate for Pasteur as had been so important with Janel. And several hospitals where we didn't have personal contacts had refused Francky's case. We decided to persist at Brigham.

"Just keep pushing," Michelle advised me. "Maybe the administration thinks you'll forget about it or give up. But just keep at it! In the end, they always do the right thing."

She was right. One day we finally received notice that we could bring one of our patients to Brigham. We chose to bring Pasteur first, given the size of his tumor and how advanced his visual deficits were. I called François and Martineau in Haiti and asked them to let Pasteur know the news and to carefully review the risks and benefits of brain surgery with him before we proceeded.

Learning from our challenges in Janel's case, we wanted Pasteur's wife to come with him to Boston so he would have someone he knew to help take care of him. Fortunately, they both had passports. And Pasteur even had a friend in Boston who offered to house him and his wife.

With housing and hospital approval in place, we got Pasteur and his wife their medical visas and booked their flights. After a long delay, things proceeded quickly.

And so, nearly two years after I'd first met Pasteur at HUM, Anne and I were waiting for him and his wife at the airport.

As dozens upon dozens of Haitian passengers flowed through customs and were received by their friends and family, I started to wonder if I had been overconfident in my promise to Anne that I'd be able to pick him out of a crowd of this size. But then, sure enough, I spotted him.

"There he is!" I called to him, "Pasteur!!"

He heard me and stopped to look around, trying to find me in his one remaining corner of vision. Pasteur kept his head and face cleanly shaven and had plump cheeks and small ears that gave him a boyish appearance. His wife, Dorotie, was taller than him and had her hair pulled back tightly. They were wrestling with two large suitcases each, all four with broken handles. Anne and I each took one as we walked toward the airport exit.

"*Kouman ou ye?*" I asked Pasteur excitedly. ("How are you?")

"*Avek Jezi!*" he declared, smiling broadly. ("With Jesus!")

"*W la!*" I said to Pasteur, smiling back at him. ("You're here!")

"*Bondye fè tou!*" he exclaimed. ("God can do anything!")

I noticed his right eye seemed to be bulging a bit. I didn't remember seeing that in Haiti a few months prior. The tumor must have grown.

We walked out of the airport into the humid July evening. Anne and I beamed at each other as we loaded their suitcases into her car. Somehow we had done it again! Pasteur and Dorotie got into the back seat, and we drove out of the airport parking lot.

Anne asked Pasteur and Dorotie how they knew Joseph, the man who would be housing them.

"Oh no, we don't know him," Dorotie said casually, looking out the window as the Boston skyline came into view.

"So you've never met?" Anne asked. We looked at each other, brows furrowed.

"No," Pasteur replied, "but it's all the same Haitian church, even in Boston. Our church is a family, so it's no problem."

Anne and I looked at each other again and shrugged. We drove on in silence.

When we arrived at Joseph's apartment building, he ran out to greet them.

"My pastor, my pastor!" he exclaimed exuberantly. "Oh wow! Oh wow!" He hugged them and grabbed their suitcases. *"Vini, vini!"* ("Come, come!") "Oh wow! *Vini, vini, vini!!"* Joseph was of medium height with a thin build and a slight hunch of his shoulders. He was bald on top with gray hair on the sides that connected to a gray beard, all just barely long enough to curl. Although I estimated he was in his early seventies, he had youthful bright eyes and seemed to dart from one place to another with the speed and light step of someone much younger. "Oh wow! Oh *wow! Vini, vini, vini, VINI!"* he said, laughing, nearly giggling, with excitement.

We entered the apartment building and crammed into its small elevator. We rode up several floors, the smells of various evening meals wafting in from each floor as we ascended.

Joseph lived in a one-bedroom apartment. He had set up his bedroom for Pasteur and Dorotie and put sheets on the couch for himself. Anne and I moved their suitcases into the bedroom and left Pasteur and Dorotie with Joseph to get some rest.

"I will walk the doctors downstairs and then give you something to eat," Joseph said to them. "You must be so hungry after this long trip!"

Joseph couldn't stop smiling as he led us back outside. "What a great night!" he said in lilting Creole-accented English. "I feel like I just got a million!!" He laughed.

"What a saint!" Anne said, as we drove away from Joseph's apartment building.

"I know! Is it some kind of great honor to house a pastor?"

"Who knows? But it's amazing to know people like him exist."

———————

The next morning I went to pick up Pasteur at Joseph's to take him for his first appointments at Brigham. Dorotie joined him. Pasteur sat with me in the front, Dorotie in the back. As we were driving, I asked Pasteur if he had any questions, hoping my Creole would be good enough to answer him.

"Will I be able to go home after the surgery?" he asked.

"You will have to stay in the hospital for at least a few days, maybe more," I said. "Then you'll have to stay in Boston while we wait to find out what type of tumor it is and whether you need other kinds of treatment. It will be at least a few weeks." I thought of how Janel had ended up spending almost a year in Boston and felt my stomach clench. "It could be longer . . ."

"Will the surgery use a laser?" he asked. It took me a few moments to understand "laser" in Creole, which is pronounced "la-*zair*." But even when I figured out what he had said, I wasn't sure what he meant. A laser? Was he referring to radiation therapy? Maybe a doctor in Haiti had mentioned that to him as a possibility.

We stopped at a red light and I looked over at him.

"No," I said. "They will have to do surgery to get the tumor out, like we discussed in Haiti." Hadn't we? Yes, I remembered us discussing how the surgery was too big and too risky to do in Haiti. Had we never made it clear that a big surgery meant opening his head? My heart sank. Did he not realize what he had signed up for? I looked out through the windshield and was glad to see the light was still red. I turned back to Pasteur.

"Because the tumor is so big, they need to cut open your head to take it out," I explained, watching for his reaction.

"Will I have a scar?" he asked, frowning, concerned.

I became concerned as well—concerned that he hadn't understood all this before he came.

"Yes, you will have a scar." I traced an arc from his right brow over his bald forehead to the closely cropped hair over his right ear with my index finger as I had seen Ian do with Janel before his surgery. "You will have a scar there."

The light turned green, and I looked away from him to begin driving. I glanced up at Dorotie in the rearview mirror. She was looking out the window in silence.

"Will I have *move kò*?" Pasteur asked me as we drove. *Move kò* literally means "bad body." I hadn't heard the expression before. I wondered if it meant something like *move san* ("bad blood"), a description of physical symptoms related to psychosocial stressors in Haiti that I had read about in one of Paul Farmer's medical anthropology articles.

"Move kò?" I repeated the words back as a question, turning to look at him as we came to a stop at another red light. I felt bad that we were discussing this in the car, but there we were.

He opened the top button of his shirt, revealing a thick raised scar on his chest. Called a keloid, this type of scarring occurs more commonly in people of African descent. He looked down and pointed to a few additional smaller keloids on his chest, which he said were from prior pimples. Then he looked back at me. "Will the scar look like that?"

"It might," I said. "It might look like that when it heals."

He looked at me for a moment, then looked forward at the dashboard, nodding his head slowly.

We sat in silence as the light turned green, and I continued driving, wondering whether we had understood each other in Haiti and whether we were understanding each other in this conversation.

"If we don't do anything, the tumor could keep growing and cause more problems," I said, breaking the silence. "But the operation has its risks, and it will certainly leave a scar."

He didn't respond.

I remembered the confusing moment when Janel had tremulously scrawled an *X* across his consent form and we all wondered what it meant. I realized that Pasteur was the first patient we'd brought to the US from Haiti with whom I could actually communicate directly. I could pose a question to him I had always wanted to ask Janel.

"*W pè?*" I asked, looking over at him as we pulled up in front of the main entrance to Brigham. ("Are you scared?")

"No!" he responded immediately and emphatically at a higher pitch than his usual soft speaking voice, his eyes wide and his lips pursed in surprise. "*M pa pè, no! Mwen avek Jezi!*" he exclaimed at the same high pitch. ("I'm not afraid, no! I'm with Jesus!") And then, growing in intensity and enunciating each word more slowly, he added, "*Tout se nan men Bondye!*" ("Everything is in the hands of God!") He smiled and pointed upward with his index finger.

He and Dorotie got out of the car to wait in front of the hospital entrance while I went to find a place to park. My thoughts were racing. Had he really not understood he was coming for a major brain surgery? Had we not communicated that clearly over the years in Haiti? If he had just realized that he'd be having open-brain surgery, was he truly unfazed—or so deeply faithful—that it seemed to barely affect him? Or was I just not understanding any of it, lost in translation between Creole and English, faith and medical science?

We were early for Pasteur's first appointment, so we went to the hospital cafeteria. We sat at a table by the window, midday summer sun streaming in. It had been two years since I first met Pasteur, and I wanted to recall the details of how his illness began and evolved. I asked him to take me back to the first symptoms.

"In first grade, I fell and hit my head," he began. A fall. Many patients in Haiti whom I had evaluated attributed their neurologic symptoms to a fall or getting hit on the head. In most cases, the event is completely unrelated. But it's not hard to imagine that in a place with no neurologists, neurologic symptoms remain mysterious, and patients search for some type of explanation, some cause and effect.

They told me the tumor had first been diagnosed by a doctor in Port-au-Prince, who told them they needed to go to Cuba for treatment. Pasteur tried to explain to me that in Cuba he had some type of laser treatment through his nose, but I couldn't fully understand him. Maybe they had tried a transsphenoidal resection: a surgical approach to the pituitary through the nose. The tumor was far too big to attempt that now, but perhaps it wasn't when he was first diagnosed. Had he mistaken the small operating scope they would have used for a laser?

"We had two treatments, but then we ran out of money," Dorotie explained, speaking in a muted, rapid-fire staccato that contrasted with Pasteur's carefully enunciated singsong voice. "They said if we wanted to continue the treatments we had to pay more money. One day I tried to go back to the hospital to stay there with him. But they said I needed to pay one thousand dollars! One thousand dollars!!" She had said the last phrases all in one breath. She stopped and sighed. "They made me stay outside! I cried and cried. I had to call my family to ask for more money."

She spoke so quickly that I had to ask her to slow down and repeat herself so I could understand her Creole.

"You need to speak more slowly for him like I do, DoDo," Pasteur told her, stretching each word out like he was talking to a child.

"I'll try, JeanJean," she replied, looking down and away.

I smiled at their pet names for each other. "Why did you have to pay if you weren't the patient?" I asked Dorotie.

"To stay with him in the hospital so long, I had to pay," she said.

"How long were you in Cuba?" I asked.

"About twenty-four days," Pasteur said.

"And do either of you speak Spanish?" I asked.

"No!" they both said together.

I remained silent, imagining them in Cuba, not knowing Spanish, not knowing anyone, having brain surgery or some sort of treatment I still didn't completely understand.

"The first treatment was twenty thousand dollars," Pasteur said. "The second one was fifteen thousand dollars."

This was all news to me. He had never mentioned this prior surgery to me when we met in Haiti, though I guess I had never asked.

"That's expensive!" I said. "How were you able to pay for it?"

"A pastor doesn't make so much money," he said, shaking his head and frowning. "Fortunately we had some insurance through the church. But we paid all of our own money, and so much of our family's money too. We had to ask everyone we knew for money."

I stared at him, horrified by the tragic story. I thought I should clarify that all of his care in Boston would be free in case there was any doubt. If he wasn't even aware that this surgery would be big enough to leave a scar, perhaps he hadn't understood that this would be nothing like his experience in Cuba. I explained that they wouldn't pay a cent of their own money, and if they needed anything, they shouldn't hesitate to ask Anne or me.

"*Le ciel prend note!*" Pasteur exclaimed, pointing his index finger upward. ("Heaven is taking note!") "I called my family in Haiti last night and said, 'They paid for our flights, they picked us up at the airport, they gave us food.' God bless Boston!" His voice was taking on a preaching melody and rhythm, each phrase more animated than the last. "It doesn't matter how you get to heaven, if it's by way of Haiti or by way of Boston! In the glory of God, amen!!" He raised his hands as if addressing his congregation.

"Amen," I said without thinking. I'm not a religious person and couldn't remember the last time I'd been in a synagogue, church, or temple aside from tourist sites when traveling. But Pasteur's slow, melodic incantations were inspiring.

"You kept coming back to HUM, and I kept telling you, 'I'm still trying,'" I said as we stood up to walk to his MRI appointment. "Others might have given up, but you didn't. And here you are."

"Louange à Dieu," he said softly. ("Praise God.")

Michelle was working at Brigham and stopped by to meet Pasteur and Dorotie in the waiting room after Pasteur's MRI while I went to look at the scan with the neuroradiologist. I had seen his enormous tumor on the CT scan he'd had at HUM, but the detail afforded by the MRI made the mass even more striking.

Several inches behind the eyes, just below the center of the brain, lies the sella turcica—literally "Turkish saddle" in Latin. In this saddle sits the pea-size pituitary gland, the endocrine command center that provides hormonal control of the thyroid, adrenal glands, and reproductive system. The optic chiasm passes just above it, transmitting the sense of sight from the eyes to the brain. Blood pulses past on either side through the carotid arteries, whose branches supply the majority of the brain's oxygen and nutrients.

Arising from Pasteur's pituitary was a fist-size tumor expanding irregularly outward in all directions, enveloping the optic chiasm above it, encasing one of the carotid arteries beside it, and indenting the adjacent brain, deforming its normal contours.

I took some pictures on my phone and sent them to Ian. We had waited over two years to see the true shape and extent of Pasteur's tumor in full detail beyond what we could see on his CT scan. I smiled when I saw Ian's characteristically short, surgical reply, reminiscent of our correspondence about Janel:

Wow, that's huge.

I came back from the radiology reading room to find Michelle beaming from ear to ear as Pasteur appeared to preach to her. *"Se doktè ki swenye, mais se Bondye ki geri!"* he was proclaiming as I arrived. ("It's the doctor who heals, but it is God who cures!")

"I'm *loving* this!" Michelle said as we walked with them outside into the afternoon sun.

"When we arrived, did you notice I was wearing a bright green shirt?" Pasteur asked us in Creole. "And my wife was wearing green too. Green is the color of hope! And this building is green!" he said, touching the wall of the hospital building we'd just emerged from.

Michelle and I hadn't heard about the significance of colors in Haiti and asked him about them.

"You don't know about the colors?!" he asked. "Red is victory, white is purity, yellow is treason, black is death. We wore green! Bright green! Hope!" He tapped against the green wall of the hospital again. *"Lespwa!"* ("Hope!")

Michelle and I couldn't stop beaming. I imagined we were both thinking the same thing: from the villages of Haiti to the medical metropolis of Boston. Our daily workplace on this hot, humid summer day transformed by Pasteur's words, creating the feeling that we might as well be chatting under a mango tree in Mirebalais.

"They are heavenly!!" Michelle texted me as I led Pasteur back inside for his next appointment. "Got my dose of church for the day!"

"Amen," I replied.

"Sometimes I think things that aren't real. Is that caused by the tumor?" Pasteur said as we sat in one of the neurosurgery clinic rooms waiting for Ian.

"Can you give me an example?" I asked him, not sure I had understood.

"There are things you can say to people and things you can't . . ." he said.

Before he could clarify, Ian entered, and Pasteur and I stood to greet him. Ian firmly and briskly shook hands with Pasteur and me and then sat down next to us in front of a large computer screen that took up nearly the entire surface of a small desk.

"I can translate," I said.

Ian nodded once without looking away from the computer screen, where he opened Pasteur's chart and began scrolling through his MRI images.

He turned to look at me. "How long did we estimate for length of stay in the hospital?" he asked, slightly under his breath.

"A week or something like that," I replied.

He looked at me a moment longer and then turned back to the computer screen and continued reviewing the MRI.

He turned back to me, expressionless. "This is a huge case," he said without breaking eye contact or blinking. He held my eyes with his for a few moments, blinked once, and then turned back to the computer. "Right up against the hypothalamus," he muttered to himself. The hypothalamus sits above the pituitary and controls it, serving as a command center for countless vital bodily functions.

Ian turned toward Pasteur and oriented him to the scans. "These are your eyes, this is your nose," he said. "And this is the tumor." He traced the tumor's irregular contour with the cursor's white arrow for Pasteur on the computer screen.

Pasteur looked at the black-and-white image for a moment and then looked at Ian. "Will there be a laser?" he asked.

"No," Ian said, looking at Pasteur. "No laser."

"Will I have a scar?" he asked, opening his shirt to show his keloids to Ian.

"Yes," Ian said. "There will be a scar."

They maintained an intense eye contact.

"It's a big surgery," Ian said soberly, directly to him. I translated.

Pasteur didn't react.

I explained to Ian that we'd been through all of this earlier in the day. I didn't want him to think I'd brought a patient to him without explaining how big a surgery this was going to be. I wondered why Pasteur was asking Ian all of the same questions he had already asked me. Were he and I not understanding each other? Was he just curious to confirm with Ian what I had told him? Or maybe it was all just overwhelming and he was trying to keep track of everything, as would be the case for any patient about to undergo brain surgery.

Ian examined him and then told him he'd see him before the surgery. He stood, smiled briefly at Pasteur, and then put out his hand. Pasteur rose slowly and shook it with both hands.

"Thank *you*!" Pasteur burst out in heavily accented English as Ian walked toward the door.

Ian stopped in the doorway and turned back to look at Pasteur.

Pasteur smiled broadly and added, again in English, "God bless *you*!"

Ian smiled back briefly, gave a quick nod, pivoted to turn down the hall, and disappeared.

"You know some English?" I asked Pasteur as we started walking out of the clinic.

He stopped, smiled softly, and shrugged. "Goood mor-neeeng!" he said. He raised his hands in front of him. "Good morneeng, my brozzers and seestersssss!" He laughed softly.

I laughed with him. Then I heard Ian's deep voice in my mind—*This is a huge case*—and stopped laughing.

We began walking through the hospital to get to the parking lot.

"What is meant by a big surgery?" Pasteur asked me as we walked.

I was glad it was starting to sink in. Based on his questions about lasers and scars, I feared I had not adequately prepared him for what lay ahead. I had never really known how much Janel understood about what was going on or whether he had truly wanted all of the medical treatment he received. It had weighed heavily on me. But here was a chance to try to do things better.

"Well, it's big for many reasons," I began. "A surgery on your thumb would be small: a small reason for it, a small incision, a quick surgery."

"Yes, it's just a little finger," he said.

"Right. But because this surgery goes into your head around your brain, it is big. Because it will take many hours, it is big. Because it will have a big scar, it is big. And because the recovery is long, it will be big."

My limited Creole forced me to speak simply, but maybe that was for the best.

He looked at me silently for a few moments and then shrugged. *"E ben, Dye konnen,"* he said ("Well, God knows"), with no more emotion than if I had told him it might rain tomorrow.

"Are you scared?" Although I had asked him this earlier that morning, I thought he understood everything more clearly now and I wanted to see how he felt.

"No, I'm not scared, no!" he said with the same intonation and facial expression as a few hours earlier. "Do you know the story of Isaac?"

"I'm not sure," I replied.

"God asked his father to sacrifice him," Pasteur explained.

"Ah, Isaac, yes, sorry," I said. Pasteur's Creole pronunciation had sounded more like "Ee-*zak*" as opposed to "*I*-saac." "Actually, I think maybe I do know that story." Somewhere out there in the universe, I imagined my second grade Sunday school teacher smiling. "Isaac and Jacob, right?"

"No, not Jacob, Abraham!" he corrected me.

The Sunday school teacher somewhere out there in the ether shook her head and frowned with disappointment.

"God asked Abraham to sacrifice his own son to test his faith," he began, "but when they arrived to do it, God produced a ram!" His voice had risen with excitement. "A ram! *Bondye ka fè tou bagay!*" he exclaimed joyfully. ("God can do anything!")

A few people walking by us in the hospital turned to look at us, the man with the bulging right eye passionately speaking in Creole to the young doctor walking beside him. Pasteur saw that he had attracted attention by speaking louder than the normal hospital din. More softly, with reverence and seriousness, he repeated, *"Bondye ka fè tou bagay."*

"So why did you think of this story when I asked if you were scared about the surgery?" I asked him.

"Because it shows God can do anything!" he said with quiet confidence, pointing one finger upward. He grinned.

We reached my car and got in. "I admire your courage," I said, before starting the car. "But it's important to understand it's a big surgery. A big brain surgery. It has risks. We hope it will help you, but it could also cause new problems for you. We don't know." I thought of Janel's vacant, wide-eyed stare and tried to suppress a shudder. "I want to make sure you understand."

"*Dye konnen ...*" he said, trailing off and looking away, nodding slowly. ("God knows.")

I started the car and began driving.

"*Glwa a letenel!*" he said with quiet passion. ("Glory to the eternal one!")

"Are you going to rest this weekend before the surgery?" I asked him.

"On Sunday Joseph is taking us to his church," Pasteur said.

"Nice," I replied. I wondered if I should ask if I could join him. I was curious to see this community that had welcomed and supported a complete stranger. And curious to witness what sounded like very high-energy church services, based on what I had heard in Haiti. There's a church across the street from the staff house in Mirebalais. Lively music, resounding sermons reaching a feverish pitch, and emphatic call-and-response often wafted into our windows late into the night.

"What do you think about me coming with you?" I asked. I felt a little guilty that it was a request made out of curiosity rather than a religiously motivated one. I didn't want to offend him.

"Of course!" he exclaimed, smiling broadly. "All are welcome!!"

"You know, I'm not Christian, so . . ." I began.

"Of course I know!" he said. "Aaron, the brother of Moses! It's a Jewish name!"

"True," I said and laughed, "but I'm not really—"

"I want everyone in the church to meet my doctor!" he said enthusiastically.

I laughed again. "I'm just a small member of a big team, Pasteur."

"God bless this team!" he intoned joyfully, raising his fists in front of him.

One by one, they emerged from Joseph's apartment building into the bright summer morning. Joseph led the way at a bouncing pace in a slightly too big black suit, white shirt, and red tie. Pasteur ambled behind in a gray checkered suit, light purple shirt embroidered with tiny purple diamond shapes, and a purple and black tie, carrying his Bible in a small leather case. Dorotie followed him in a black dress patterned with a red and green floral print around the neck and sleeves, her hair pulled back tightly with a barrette adorned with a large black flower.

I exchanged kisses on each cheek with Dorotie and shook hands with Joseph and Pasteur. Pasteur's handshake was gentle and welcoming, his hand slightly pudgy. I smiled at him. Then I heard Ian's voice in my head: *This is a huge case.* Pasteur and Dorotie looked so happy to be going to church, but I couldn't help feeling a certain sadness and trepidation. What if Pasteur's case turned out to be a long drawn-out saga like Janel's? No, I tried to reassure myself as we got into Joseph's car, he was starting from a much better place than Janel. Still, that meant he had further to fall. I hoped he would make it out of this unscathed.

As we entered the church, I felt like I had walked through a secret portal directly into Haiti. Everyone inside was Haitian, speaking in Creole. Women wore broad-brimmed church hats with various combinations of fancy buckles, sequins, and lace. Older men wore oversize somber dark suits and dull primary-colored ties that dangled below their waists. Younger men wore tight gray or white suits, brightly colored shirts, and fashionable patterned ties. A band composed of organ, guitar, bass, and drums was tuning their instruments. Joseph excitedly introduced me to people as we took our place in one of the front pews.

The service began with the minister introducing guests from outside the congregation who were attending the service. Amid the list of Haitian names, I heard my name.

"Stand up," Joseph whispered to me.

I stood for a moment, then began to sit back down.

"No, stay standing!" the pastor said to me in Creole.

I stood back up and smiled apologetically.

"Ah! He smiled!" the pastor continued in Creole and laughed. "You see this Jewish man visiting us speaks Creole, French, English." Then in Creole-inflected English he said, "We are glad you are here, and you must return, each Sabbath! Every Sabbath!! We save that seat for you!"

I blushed in the heat of many eyes looking at me and sat down.

The melodies, harmonies, and rhythms of the liturgy sounded similar to what I'd heard walking past churches in Haiti, a combination of chorale and Caribbean. So did the impassioned "Amens" that careened frequently through the congregation.

The pastor delivering the sermon was tall and heavyset, his shaved head making his plump face look like a perfect circle floating above his flowing black tunic. The sermon he delivered was in a style I'd become familiar with in Haiti through the blaring loudspeakers of the church across from the staff house in Mirebalais. With each paragraph, the preacher's phrases increased progressively in volume and intensity, culminating in a throat-tearing, speaker-crackling raspiness, only to give way suddenly to a quiet statement, a question, or a pause and a laugh before starting a similar crescendo to another peak of frenzied screaming. Microphone after microphone gave out, and someone ran over to the pulpit to provide a freshly charged one. The batteries must be dying because it is such hard work keeping up with the intensity of preaching, I thought.

The pastor preached in very fast Creole, and I would have been completely lost if there hadn't been a large screen displaying a PowerPoint presentation of key phrases and images, like those out of a Sunday school children's book. The sermon discussed "Deliverance du Feu" ("Deliverance from the Fire")—Daniel, chapter 3. From what I could understand of the PowerPoint and bits of Creole I caught, three men were thrown into a fire for refusing to pray to idols, but Jesus saved them. At the preacher's speaker-distorting climax, he nearly screamed, each phrase incanted faster than the previous. "They should have burned, but they didn't! They should have burned, but Jesus was there! They should have burned, but they were saved!! Saved for doing what was right!! Saved because Jesus was there!!! Jesus saved them!!! Saved them from the fire!!!! Saved!!!! From the fire!!!! Saved by *Jesus*!!!!!!"

He paused.

Silence.

And then in a soft, conversational, deep voice, "God made the fire feel like air-conditioning for them." He chuckled.

I looked over at Pasteur. His eyes were closed. Was he sleeping? Meditating? Praying? He usually spoke so softly and slowly, and I found it hard to imagine that he would preach in this style of accelerating screams. I wanted to remember to ask him later.

The man who appeared to be the head priest called Pasteur to the altar and asked Dorotie, Joseph, and me to join the group of clergy and senior members of the church who had assembled on the stage. Pasteur stumbled and nearly fell climbing the stairs to the raised platform behind the pulpit and was caught by some of the nearby clergy. "Be careful," the priest said solemnly to him. Suddenly I felt nervous. *What if he had fallen? What if he had fallen and had a seizure?* I thought.

The priest explained to the congregation that Pasteur was visiting from Haiti for a large surgery *nan tèt li* (inside his head). There were gasps and whispers. The priest explained that I was one of Pasteur's doctors. He asked the congregation for their prayers for Pasteur, for his surgery, and for his surgeon. They guided Pasteur, Dorotie, Joseph, and me to the center of the sanctuary, just behind the lectern, and asked Pasteur and Dorotie to kneel. I thought someone signaled me to do so as well. But as I started to lower myself down, someone else said in a harsh whisper in Creole, "No, not you. Stand up!" I already felt out of place in a church, let alone being the only non-Haitian person in a

Haitian church, and now I felt even more awkward to be up there with them.

The group made a circle around Pasteur and Dorotie and held hands. A smaller group, including Joseph, stood inside the circle next to Pasteur, each putting a hand on his shoulder or Dorotie's. I wasn't sure whether to hold hands with the outer circle or put my hand on Pasteur's shoulder with the inner circle. I wanted to participate if they wanted me to but not intrude or offend anyone after my confusion about whether I was supposed to kneel or stand. The people on either side of me took my hands, and so I became part of the outer circle.

One priest knelt facing the congregation, his back to us, leading songs and prayers. Members of the congregation swayed as they sang, some with their hands reaching up toward the ceiling above, waving slowly. One of the priests directly across from me in the circle rocked gently, eyes closed, smiling serenely, softly murmuring occasional phrases like "Amen" and *"Jezi la"* ("Jesus is here"). I looked at Pasteur and Dorotie. With many hands on their shoulders, their eyes gently closed, they looked at peace.

I was grateful to see them welcomed into this community. I hoped the benediction would be meaningful for them, a feeling of home despite being so far away from Haiti. But Pasteur's near fall up the stairs troubled me. As I looked at him, despite the soothing, slow melodies intoned by the priest and congregation, my mind raced with anxious thoughts. *What if he has a seizure right here, right now?* It wasn't rational. He had never had a seizure, though he was certainly at risk for one. Why would he have one now? Was I remembering that Janel had had one of his seizures in church?

My thoughts wandered to a piano recital I had attended nearly twenty years earlier. A cameraman filming the concert from a raised platform fainted and slowly slumped over in plain view of the audience. Proceeding like a silent film, there was a quiet, hushed sense of alarm as paramedics carried the limp, ailing man out of the concert hall to the soundtrack of the pianist's melancholic Chopin, which continued in spite of the calm commotion. The pianist must have been bewildered if he noticed that the audience members kept turning their heads toward the back corner of the concert hall. Or maybe he could make out the action out of the corner of his eye. Did he ask himself whether he should stop playing or just continue with his concert? Somehow he had kept playing. I hadn't thought about that surreal moment in years.

I imagined a similar situation here if Pasteur suddenly had a seizure. Quiet panic behind the pulpit as the music went on for the congregation. Nothing to see here. *Please don't let him have a seizure, please don't let him have a seizure, please don't let him have a seizure,* I thought over and over. *This must be my way of trying to pray as a neurologist,* I tried to joke to myself. *This is a huge case,* I heard Ian's deep voice intone in response.

Despite my internal agitation, the scene in front of me was deeply moving. Hands in hands and hands on shoulders and hands slowly swaying in the air, catching rays of colored light from the sun streaming through the stained-glass windows. A single verse of the last hymn, sung more softly and slowly with each repetition. And Pasteur and Dorotie at the center, eyes closed, soft smiles, welcomed, embraced, blessed.

This part of the ceremony ended, and we filed down the stairs back to our pew. As I passed one of the priests, he took my hand in his, looked into my eyes, and put his other hand over our hands. "Thank you, Doctor," he said in strongly accented English. "And please return to our church. Please return."

When it came time for the children's part of the service, I asked Joseph if he could tell me where the bathroom was. He offered to take me. We'd been there for over three hours, so I supposed he needed a break too. After we left the bathroom, I took advantage of this being the first time I was alone with him.

"Joseph, do you think Pasteur understands the surgery?"

"Oh yes," he said. "This pastor has had many members of the church who have had surgery."

"Ah no," I replied. "Not the church's pastor, I mean *our* Pasteur, Jean-Rémy."

"Oh," he said, and he led me outside to the front steps of the church.

"I want to make sure he really understands," I said. "This is a big surgery, and it has risks."

"I think he does understand," he said calmly. "We talk about it and pray together."

"If he doesn't have surgery, the tumor will progress. He could become fully blind."

"He could even die," Joseph replied, anticipating my next words.

"But the surgery . . . it's risky. He could have problems after it that he doesn't have now."

"There, too, he could even die," Joseph said matter-of-factly.

"Do you think he and his wife understand this?" I asked. "I've explained it to them, but there can be miscommunications with the language barrier and the cultural differences. Pasteur even asked me whether he would have a scar, so I wondered if he really understood the magnitude of all this."

"I think he does," Joseph said reassuringly. "But we will keep talking about it."

"He doesn't seem afraid . . ." I began.

"No, he's not," he replied, flashing a smile.

"And so I don't know if that's because he doesn't fully understand the magnitude of this or just because he has such faith or—"

"It's his faith!" he interrupted emphatically. "As Christians, we believe God can do anything, so we don't need to be afraid." He laughed gently.

Like Jesus turning the fire into air-conditioning, I thought.

We went back inside.

"We pray for one of our church elders who will have surgery in the spine," the pastor was saying as we sat down. There were some gasps in the congregation. "It's a big surgery, but we're not worried. *Bondye ka fè tou bagay!*" ("God can do anything!") "We pray for her! And when is Pasteur Jean-Rémy's surgery?" he asked in Creole. Then, looking at me in the third pew, he switched to English. "Monday?"

"Tuesday," I replied.

"We pray for him!" he proclaimed.

"Amen," the congregation replied in impassioned unison.

On the drive home, Pasteur said, "I met a lady who told me she had a tumor like me. She was going blind too. And then she was cured!"

"She had surgery like you will have?" I asked.

"No!" Pasteur said. "It went away on its own!"

"A miracle," Joseph said, smiling and nodding.

Then he turned to me. "But I don't believe it," he said in English and laughed. "Must have been something else. Tumors don't just go away like that." He laughed again.

I laughed too. *I guess faith has its limits*, I thought.

"Pasteur, do you preach like that?" I asked, turning around from the front seat to look at him. "Screaming into the microphone?"

"Yes!" he said, grinning and raising one fist in front of his chest.

"But you normally speak so softly and gently."

"Preaching is different than talking!" he said, shaking the fist in front of his chest.

Joseph dropped Pasteur and Dorotie off at his apartment and offered to drive me home. He pulled up outside my apartment building, and I thanked him for welcoming me into their church.

"You see, our church is like this worldwide," he said. "Anywhere you go—Haiti, Africa, Boston—we are a family. You are welcome there. Everyone is welcome there!" He smiled warmly. *"Lè ou pa gen fanmi, se legliz ki fanmi w,"* he said and laughed. "You understand?"

I thought about it for a moment. "When you don't have family, the church is your family," I said and smiled.

"Wow, you really understand Creole!" He chuckled, patting my shoulder.

"You're a real saint," I said as I got out of his car. "I really appreciate all you've done to make Pasteur feel so at home."

It was indeed amazing to see Pasteur absorbed into this community, as if despite the short drive from Boston we had somehow spent the morning in the warm, welcoming, worshipping world of Haiti. I thought back to Janel's time in Boston, isolated and alone, fighting with the group of older women who had tried to take care of him. I winced. We were certainly doing better this time at making our patient feel at home. But somehow I spent the rest of the day feeling uneasy. Maybe it was seeing Pasteur and his wife so content when they received their blessing while my mind raced with the odd fear that he could have a seizure in the church. Or maybe it was the accumulation of instances in which his soft-spoken, smiling greeting and smooth, plump handshake had become juxtaposed in my mind with Ian's sober neurosurgical assessment: *This is a huge case.*

What if the surgery left him with a paralyzed limb, cognitive difficulties, or a seizure disorder? What if he ended up with chronic pituitary dysfunction requiring advanced endocrine management and monitoring that we couldn't take care of in Haiti? All were possible outcomes. But if he didn't have surgery, many of these were possible outcomes too, as was losing his last sliver of sight and becoming fully blind, the very outcome we were trying to prevent. And yet things had progressed so slowly over time. He hadn't lost any more vision in the two years that I had known him. Perhaps he would have five more good years, or more, before anything got worse. It was hard to know. But he could wake up from the surgery a very different person from who he was before. Instantly.

The weight of it felt immense. In my day-to-day practice as a neurologist I never have the feeling of playing God that I imagine some surgeons experience when they operate at the acute frontiers of life and death. Yet with Janel, with Davidson, and now with Pasteur, even though I wasn't going to hold the scalpel, I felt responsible for bringing them to the scalpel and, in so doing, for tinkering with the natural order of things.

Of course there is nothing natural about an order of things in which Pasteur's tumor had left him nearly blind and had grown to become a *huge case*, when it could have been identified and treated years earlier if he hadn't been born in Haiti with no access to basic healthcare, let alone advanced healthcare. In fact, it's quite an *un*natural world order where the poorest suffer, become disabled, and die of diseases that are easily treated elsewhere.

It's rare that I ever think I might be able to make a meaningful dent, however small, in these steep gradients of inequity. Most of the time my work feels like a small drop in a big bucket, a bucket with a huge hole at the bottom. Or maybe no bottom at all. Although trying to help an individual patient like Pasteur gave me the sense of a certain immediacy of impact, it also seemed fraught with countless risks and complexities. Objectively, his tumor was large and it was growing—I couldn't stand aside and do nothing. And yet doing something could have grave consequences. Janel hadn't recovered much from his five surgeries. It was possible he never would.

I was clearly more worried about all of this than Pasteur was. For him, a woman in the congregation could have her tumor cured by a miracle, and three men could be thrown into a fire and come out unscathed. It just required faith.

———————

I walked through the preoperative area at Brigham along rows of gurneys separated by tan checkered curtains. When I found Pasteur's bed, he was already dressed in a blue-and-white checkered hospital gown. A nurse was placing an IV in his left arm. Dorotie was standing at his bedside in an orange T-shirt and denim skirt, and Anne and

Joseph stood on either side of her. I said hi to Anne and then greeted Pasteur, Joseph, and Dorotie, asking, *"Kouman ou ye?"* ("How are you?") to each in turn.

"Avek Jezi," Pasteur replied softly but firmly. ("With Jesus.")

"Anfom," said Joseph calmly. ("Fine.")

When I turned to Dorotie, she looked away and began softly sobbing.

Joseph smiled at her and said, "Don't do that, don't do that. Everything will be okay."

Anne put her arm around Dorotie's shoulders and led her outside the small curtained-off area.

Joseph and I lingered next to Pasteur's bed but didn't speak.

The anesthesia team arrived to put an arterial line in Pasteur's wrist under sterile conditions and sent Joseph and me outside the curtain. We found Anne standing in front of Dorotie, holding both of her hands, speaking softly to her as she sobbed. Anne let go of Dorotie's hands and told us she needed to leave to get to the wards to start her workday. She turned back to Dorotie, hugged her, then tenderly put her palms on Dorotie's cheeks before turning to go.

The anesthesia team finished their procedure, and we stepped back inside the curtain.

Ian's assisting neurosurgery resident came, made brief small talk with Pasteur, and then drew an *X* over his right eyebrow with a purple marker—standard practice to make sure the team operated on the correct side. I thought back to the confusing moment when Janel had scrawled an *X* on the signature line of his consent form. Things were certainly going much more smoothly with Pasteur so far. So far.

Pasteur looked at me, bent his arm, and made a fist in front of his chest. *"Viktwa!"* he said. ("Victory!")

"Rouge!" I responded and smiled, remembering he'd taught me that red was the color for victory in some Haitian tradition I still didn't really understand.

He smiled back. *"Rouge! Viktwa!"* he said again, making the same gesture with his fist.

Then we stood in silence around him. Through an opening in the curtain, I saw the patients on gurneys being rolled past one by one like floats in some strange parade, disappearing behind white double doors marked by a red stop sign reading:

RESTRICTED ACCESS

STAFF ONLY

Ian emerged from these double doors and came into the curtained area, appearing laser-focused as always. He greeted everyone with a wave and a brief smile. "I'll see you in back," he told Pasteur. Then he turned and stepped out of the curtained area and I followed him.

"This is going to be a long case," he said to me calmly and quietly in his deep voice. "There are two main aspects of this operation that are dangerous: vascular injury and capsular bleeding."

Vascular injury I understood: the carotid artery was encased by the tumor. If the artery was irritated or damaged during the surgery, this could lead to a stroke. I wasn't familiar with his second concern. "Capsular bleeding?" I asked.

"You've got to stay inside the tumor capsule," he said matter-of-factly, looking to the right of me, then back at me. "Otherwise you risk major bleeding."

I nodded, trying to imagine him mentally preparing to stay inside the several-centimeter space of the tumor capsule for the next ten or more hours.

"I'm going to go in back and set up," he said. "The nurse will text you with updates." He turned and walked with his confident surgeon's stride—slightly hunched upper back; long, quick steps—toward the white swinging doors with the red stop sign, pushed through them, and disappeared.

I stepped back inside the tan curtain.

"We're going to go back now," the nurse said to Dorotie and Joseph. "Time for hugs and kisses!" She smiled.

Dorotie stood frozen, looking anxiously at Pasteur.

"Go give him a kiss," Joseph said to her and chuckled.

Dorotie hesitated. Then she leaned forward and timidly kissed his forehead the way a child might kiss her elderly grandfather goodbye after being forced to do so by her parents. She started sobbing again and walked outside the curtain, covering her face.

"Don't do that, don't do that," Joseph gently scolded, following her.

"It's okay," I said, stepping out with them.

A clicking sound marked the unlocking of the wheels of Pasteur's gurney. Then the curtain opened and the nurse wheeled him toward us.

The nurse stopped in front of us, and I shook his hand. "*W nan bon men,*" I said. ("You're in good hands.")

"*Men Jezi!*" he said with quiet passion. ("The hands of Jesus!") A single tear sprang from his bulging right eye and trickled slowly down his cheek. As the nurse pushed his gurney past us, he raised his fist in front of his chest again, and Joseph and I did the same.

As soon as he was out of sight, Dorotie burst out crying more forcefully. Joseph put his arm around her as we walked out.

I left them to go to my clinic, already late, wondering how I was going to focus on the patients I would see that day knowing that Pasteur was under the knife, remembering how terrible Janel had looked after his first surgery.

As I saw my patients in the neurology clinic, I got updates on my pager throughout the day that the operation was "going okay."

Then, for several hours, I heard nothing.

Four p.m. passed.

Five p.m. passed.

I paged Ian's assistant and asked if she had any updates.

"The status in the electronic operative record is 'Closing,'" she said, "so they must be almost done."

I couldn't take the suspense and called the operating room myself. The operating room nurse who answered said that the surgery was finished and they were about to try to wake the patient up.

I waited for a text from Ian.

Finally, at 5:30 p.m., one arrived.

> Ian: All done, waiting for wake up.
>
> Me: Thanks. How'd it go?
>
> Ian: It went well. Very tough case—tumor is so extensive. There are capsular remnants and tumor in sella and around carotid but I think we accomplished the goal. Main risk now is bleeding.
>
> Me: I will update his family. When do you think OK to tell them to come see him? 1–1.5 hours?
>
> Ian: I think. His right eye will be swollen. He will maybe not be wide awake.
>
> Me: Got it and will relay.

About ten minutes later:

> Ian: Slow to wake up so getting CT, but not too unusual.
>
> Me: Got it. Thanks.

About five minutes later:

> Ian: CT is fine. He may stay intubated overnight.

I called Joseph to let him know the surgery was over and all had gone well, but Pasteur was still asleep and on the breathing machine. I asked him if Dorotie wanted to come see him.

"No, no, she doesn't want to see him tonight," he said. "We will come tomorrow."

"I'll see you then," I said.

The next morning, I took the elevator up to the neuro-ICU to see Pasteur before Dorotie and Joseph arrived. Reading the nurses' notes on my phone on the way up, I saw that he had been extubated (they had taken the breathing tube out) and he was following commands (able to understand what others said to him). These were all promising signs that everything had gone well. I breathed a sigh of relief as the elevator ascended.

I entered the neuro-ICU and walked around the arc of patient rooms until I saw Pasteur. His head was tightly wrapped in a turban of white gauze. The region around his right eye was grotesquely swollen as though he'd been in a bad fight, the eyelid so puffy it sealed his eye shut. He was asleep.

"Pasteur?" I said.

"*Wi . . .*" he responded lethargically, his eyes closed. ("Yes . . .")

"*Pasteur, se Doktè Aaron!*" ("Pasteur, it's Dr. Aaron.")

"*Wi . . .*" He opened his left eye and reached out his right hand to shake mine.

"*Pasteur, kouman ou ye?*" ("Pasteur, how are you?")

"*A-a-a-a-a-an-fom,*" he stuttered. ("O-o-o-o-o-o-kay.")

Why was he stuttering? The surgery had been on the right side of his brain, and language is almost always controlled by the left side of the brain.

"*Pasteur, kouman madam ou rele?*" I asked him. ("Pasteur, what is your wife's name?")

"Do-do-do-do-do-do-rotie," he stuttered rhythmically.

I cursed.

His nurse came in and asked him if he needed anything.

"*Agua,*" he said. I didn't know he spoke any Spanish.

His nurse tried to give him a sip of water, and it all spilled down his chin onto his gown, making an expanding dark spot.

As I observed him, I noticed he was moving his right arm and leg but not his left arm or leg.

"*Pasteur, leve men goch.*" ("Pasteur, lift up your left hand.")

He raised his right hand but didn't move the left. I put my hand in his left hand.

"*Kenbe men'm, Pasteur.*" ("Squeeze my hand, Pasteur.")

He reached up his right hand and groped the air, but his left hand remained lifeless in mine.

I gave him a brief pinch on his left hand, and he briskly pulled it away. He could move it, so that was good, but he didn't wince to indicate that he noticed the pain.

I cursed again.

He had developed a neurologic problem called neglect.

With problems on the left side of the brain that paralyze the right side of the body, patients are almost always very aware that they are paralyzed on the right. But with problems on the right side of the brain that paralyze the left side of the body, many patients develop neglect—they ignore the paralyzed left side, not seeming to notice that it's weak. In extreme cases, patients with neglect don't even recognize the left side of their body as their own. Once I showed a patient with neglect her left hand and asked her whose hand it was. "That's your hand," she said with complete confidence. I pointed out to her that the hand in front of her had her wedding ring on it. "How did you get my wedding ring!?" she asked me with shock and anger.

Pasteur's tumor had encased the carotid artery on the right side. The right carotid artery provides most of the blood supply to the right hemisphere of the brain. Could the artery have been damaged during the operation and caused a stroke?

And what was with the stuttering? I tried to tell myself not to worry about Pasteur's deficits until I spoke with Ian—maybe Pasteur's right hemisphere was just stunned in some way from being retracted for several hours so Ian could operate beneath it. I worried nevertheless. If Pasteur couldn't speak properly and couldn't move his left side, it was hard to imagine him returning to his life as a pastor. I was afraid things were going more in the Janel direction than the Davidson direction.

Joseph called to say he was parking the car outside Brigham, and he and Dorotie would be up soon. I met them at the elevators.

"*Kouman ou ye?*" I asked Dorotie. ("How are you?")

"*Mwen anfom, wi,*" she said. ("I'm fine.") She looked much more relaxed than the day before.

"*Mye pase yè?*" I asked. ("Better than yesterday?")

"*Wi!*" she said emphatically. "*Yè tèt mwen te gwo!*" she said in her usual rapid-fire cadence. It took me a moment to process the Creole. I thought she had said "Yesterday my head was big!"

"*Tèt ou te gwo?*" I asked, to clarify. ("Your head was big?")

"*Wi, tèt mwen te gwo,*" she repeated slightly less quickly. ("Yes, my head was big.")

I had understood the Creole but didn't understand the expression.

She smiled at my confusion. "*M te gen anpil bagay nan tèt,*" she explained. ("I had so many things in my head [on my mind].")

I added it to my collection of *tèt* (head) expressions, alongside *tèt chaje.*

As we walked, I told them that Pasteur was still waking up, so his talking was a little funny. I explained that his right eye and face were swollen but that this would get better over time. I described the large bandage wrapped around his head. I didn't want Dorotie to be frightened by how he looked. I decided not to mention that he might be neglecting his left side until I heard from Ian whether this was worrisome or some expected postoperative issue that would resolve.

I swiped my badge at the entrance to the neuro-ICU, and the automatic doors flung open. I led Dorotie and Joseph past the front desk to Pasteur's room and introduced them to his nurse.

The nurse smiled at Dorotie. "You're beautiful!" she said.

"*Li di ou bel!*" I translated for Dorotie. ("She says you're beautiful!")

Dorotie smiled nervously, looking past her at Pasteur.

She and Joseph approached his bed. "*Pasteur, cheri ou la!*" Joseph said with his usual vibrant energy. ("Pasteur, your dear wife is here!")

Pasteur opened his left eye and reached out his right hand. Dorotie took it gently, timidly, as if it were her first time holding hands with him.

"My wife," Pasteur said in English.

"Wow, wow!" Joseph exclaimed, smiling. "Already moving around and recognizing her! I thought he'd be much worse today! Wow, wow, wow! It's a miracle!"

With the head wrap, his eye swollen shut, and Pasteur being just barely awake, I had been worried they'd be disappointed if not downright frightened. But they seemed happy.

"I worked in maintenance in hospitals for thirty years," Joseph said. "I know how bad they can look after surgery! Wow!"

Dorotie stood next to Pasteur's bed, looking him over. She gently patted his knee. We brought her a chair, and she sat down beside him.

"*M ka pran foto?*" she asked me, taking out her phone. ("Can I take a picture?")

"*Foto?*" I asked. ("A picture?")

"*Wi, pou paren li. L'ap mande kouman li ye.*" ("Yes, for his family. They're asking how he is.")

She took two pictures and looked at them, smiling broadly.

I was surprised that she was so comfortable with him looking the way he did that she'd want a picture.

Li la, I thought—he's here. I remembered how Janel's mother had been so happy just to see him survive his surgeries even when we thought he looked his worst.

Later that day, I ran into Ian and mentioned that I was worried that Pasteur had developed stuttering and neglect since the surgery. "Give him time," he said. "It was a huge case." He smiled at my impatience and concern. "He'll come around."

"Yes, I remember you used to say that for Janel..." I said, trailing off. Janel did come around from his low point after surgery, but not as much as we had hoped. And then he declined again. The surgeries had gone perfectly, but maybe it had just been too late.

"Oh man, Janel!" he said and shook his head. "Every day on rounds I said, 'He'll come around,' and everyone rolled their eyes at me. But when you're the one who was in there, you know you didn't violate anything. You didn't violate any vascular structures. You didn't violate the thalamus. The brain is okay. Look, Janel's brain went from this"—he tangled his arms around each other like a pretzel—"to this." He popped his arms untangled and smiled. "Compared to Janel, this case . . ." He trailed off.

"Janel's was a big tumor," he said, looking beyond me slightly wistfully. "The biggest tumor I've ever operated on."

17

After walking about fifty steps on the main dirt road leading away from HUM, Martineau and I turned onto a small path that led off to the right. To our left was an eight-foot-high wall of gray cinder blocks topped with rings of barbed wire. To our right, a few one-room and two-room tin-roofed concrete houses about the same height as the wall. Our ankles twisted over white and gray rocks with dark green weeds sprouting between them, the path strewn with scattered trash—small pink-striped plastic bags, small blue plastic bags, and a few faded, crushed plastic soda bottles. Toward the end of the path, I spotted Janel's mother coming from behind one of the houses carrying a pink laundry basket filled with bedsheets.

She saw Martineau and me walking toward her, smiled broadly, and put down the laundry basket.

"Oooo-eee! Doktè Martineau! Doktè Aaron!" she called out.

She ran toward us and hugged each of us in turn, her thin, bony arms strong and affectionate.

We exchanged greetings as she led us up three concrete stairs to a small porch, where a shirtless, muscular young man sat working on an outdoor sewing machine. She led us past him to an unpainted, unfinished wooden door and slipped her flip-flops off her callused feet as she opened it. I reached down to remove my shoes, but she smiled and waved her hand back and forth. *"No, no—pa gen pwoblem, Dok,"* she said, gesturing excitedly for us to enter. ("No, no—no problem, Doc.")

Inside their one-room house it was dim and a few degrees cooler. The walls were painted a soft lime green. The front wall had two tombstone-shaped window openings fitted with iron grates and covered with thin, translucent pink curtains, but no windows or screens. A single non-functioning lightbulb hung on a wire from one of the wooden beams running beneath the flat tin roof. Most of the concrete floor was taken up by two mattresses, one against the far wall, the other just next to it in the center of the room. In one corner sat a few plastic bins filled with clothes and cleaning supplies. In another, a tall black suitcase, its handle hanging off like a loose tooth. Janel's mother unstacked two white plastic lawn chairs, set them out, and motioned for us to sit.

Then she went to wake Janel, who was fast asleep on the mattress in the middle of the room.

Martineau and I told her she didn't need to wake him up.

She squatted on the edge of his mattress, pulling the back of her skirt up through her legs. She smiled up at us.

"*E ben m kontan we w,*" she said. ("Well, I'm happy to see you.")

I heard rustling and a high-pitched chirping sound from the far corner of the room and turned my head just in time to see a large rat dart between the large suitcase and one of the bins along the wall. Nobody else seemed to notice, or if they did, it didn't seem to bother them.

"*Kouman Janel ye?*" Martineau asked her. ("How is Janel?")

"*L'ap mache!*" she said proudly. ("He's walking!")

She told us that she was happy with Janel's progress. Then Martineau asked her how she was.

"*E ben, n'ap lite, n'ap fè efò,*" she said. ("Well, we're struggling, we're making an effort.") It is one of many less-than-positive ways of responding to "How are you?" in Creole, not necessarily meant to be taken literally. But in her case it was true.

She explained to us that she was grateful to be receiving her monthly stipend from HUM and couldn't survive without it. But unfortunately, it usually didn't last the whole month. She told us how she wished she might save enough money to invest in *ti komers* (a little commerce), buying some goods and selling them in front of the hospital. Then she could have a self-sustaining income. But the current stipend was too little to do that.

"*M kalkile, m kalkile,*" she lamented, shaking her head. ("I'm calculating, I'm calculating.")

Martineau and I nodded somberly.

Martineau assured her he would talk with the social workers at HUM to see what might be possible to help her.

She extended her long arms out to her sides with her palms up and sighed. "*E ben, lè Bondye ba'w yon peine, li ba'w sekou apre,*" she said.

I didn't understand her. I looked at Martineau, squinted, and cocked my head to the side.

He thought for a moment and then translated, "She said, 'When God gives you a punishment, he gives you relief afterward.'" He looked down at the floor and then back at her, his expression somewhere between a wince and a smile.

A chicken clucked excitedly outside and then was drowned out by the mechanical sputtering of the sewing machine. A rooster squawked. Inside the small, dim room, we sat in silence.

Janel rolled slowly from his side onto his back. He yawned long and deep, his head shaking a little. Then he slowly sat up, facing Martineau and me in our plastic lawn chairs at the foot of his mattress. He was wearing black gym shorts and a white ribbed tank top, frayed at the edges, a hole under the right shoulder with torn threads running across it. He stared at us, his usual wide-eyed expressionless stare.

"*Bonjou, Janel,*" Martineau said. ("Hi, Janel.")

He blinked once, slowly.

"*W sonje'm, Janel?*" I asked him, leaning toward him. ("Do you remember me, Janel?")

No response.

"*Salye doktè yo, Ja!*" His mom prodded him, smiling. ("Say hi to the doctors, Ja!")

He simultaneously nodded his chin briskly upward and raised and lowered his eyebrows.

"Kouman ou ye, Janel?" I asked him. ("How are you, Janel?")

He slowly brought his right palm to his forehead, closed his eyes, and winced. Then he opened his eyes to look at Martineau and me to see if we had understood the gesture.

"W gen tèt fè mal, Janel?" Martineau asked him. ("You have a headache, Janel?")

He didn't respond. He looked at us for a few moments, then slowly raised his right hand to chin level. He formed a fist, and then made a quick, small, sharp circle in front of his chin. Then a second circle. Then a third.

Martineau and I looked at each other and then turned back to Janel. We didn't understand the gesture.

Janel kept his fist clenched in front of his chin. Then he made another series of three quick, sharp circles.

"Li ka pale?" I asked Janel's mom. ("Can he talk?")

"Wi, li kapab," she said. ("Yes, he can.") *"Pale ak doktè yo, Janel!"* she said to him. ("Talk to the doctors, Janel!")

He remained silent and made the brisk fist circles again.

Martineau and I looked at him quizzically.

He stared at us for a while. Then he slowly squeaked out a hoarse, raspy, high-pitched, two-word sentence: *"Tèt vire."* ("Head spinning.") Creole for dizziness.

"W gen tèt vire, Janel?" Martineau asked him. ("Are you dizzy, Janel?")

Janel made the fist circles again.

"All day! Mm!" his mother said emphatically, slapping the back of one hand into the palm of the other. "Some days he lies in bed all day because he says his head is spinning so much!" She shook her head.

Martineau and I discussed the possibilities. Was this just a residual symptom from his extensive surgeries? A side effect of his anti-seizure medication? Something non-neurologic, like dehydration or anemia?

While we conferred, Janel's mother rummaged through some of the bins in the corner of the room where I had seen the large rat moments before. She returned with a toothbrush, toothpaste, a plastic bottle of water, and a small basin. She put toothpaste on the toothbrush and handed it to Janel. He brushed his teeth slowly and methodically for a long time, pausing occasionally to spit thick, foamy saliva into the basin, which his mother held out in front of him.

Martineau had to go back to the hospital. He said goodbye and told me we would talk later.

After Janel finished brushing his teeth, his mother produced a small rag and a slightly larger one from the suitcase in the corner, a bar of soap from one of the corner bins, and a yellow plastic bucket of water. She wet the smaller rag in the bucket, then rubbed it vigorously on the bar of soap until it was foaming with suds. She sat facing Janel and began scrubbing his face with the rag. Janel closed his eyes as she lathered every inch of his forehead, cheeks, nose, and chin.

"*Ouvri bouch ou,*" she told him. ("Open your mouth.")

He let his jaw hang slack. She cleaned his lips. Then she moistened the second rag and gently but firmly wiped the soapsuds off his face.

There was something meditative about watching them quietly go about their routine. Janel's mother's tender and meticulous cleaning of her son's face, the soft sound of the rag scrubbing back and forth, Janel's placid acceptance of this ritual.

Janel's mother took a towel and dried his face. He kept his eyes gently closed. Then he opened them again. His mother walked to the corner of the room to put her toiletries away.

I asked Janel if I could examine him to figure out why he was dizzy. He didn't reply.

"*Swivi dwet mwen ak zye w,*" I said, moving my index finger back and forth in front of his eyes. ("Follow my finger with your eyes.") He did this perfectly. I was looking for nystagmus, a jerking movement of the eyes that can be seen when anti-seizure medications reach toxic doses, or with problems of the cerebellum or vestibular system. He didn't have any nystagmus, so the problem was probably not his medications or an active problem in the back of his brain where part of his tumor had been.

"*Eske ou ka touche dwet mwen ak dwet ou epi touche nen ou apre?*" I asked. ("Can you touch my finger with your finger and then touch your nose?") This test examines coordination. He did it perfectly, without any of the trembling incoordination he'd had before his surgeries.

"*M ka we ou mache?*" I asked him. ("Can I see you walk?")

He didn't respond.

"*Fè yon ti mache pou doktè a!*" his mom called excitedly from the corner. ("Do a little walking for the doctor!")

He moved his fist in small, sharp, rapid circles again—the dizzy symbol.

"*W gen tèt vire la kounyea?*" I asked him. ("Are you feeling dizzy right now?")

He made the gesture again.

"*An nou mache, Ja!*" his mother encouraged him. ("Come on, let's walk, Ja!") She was standing above him now and reached out her hand.

Janel shook his head and lifted one hand in a stop gesture. His mom withdrew her hand and smiled at him.

He sat quietly, staring forward. After a few moments, he slowly scooted himself to the edge of the mattress. He paused. Then he leaned his torso forward over his knees. He paused again. Carefully, holding his arms slightly out to his sides, he gradually straightened his legs, his torso still bent slightly forward. He paused in this position. Finally, still in slow motion, he lifted his torso and then his head, as if stacking each bone of his spine one on top of the next. And then he was standing. I had forgotten how tall he was, having mostly seen him lying in a hospital bed. He towered head and shoulders above his mother. He stood there, not moving, his feet spread slightly wider than his hips. I thought of a young child standing for the first time, not taking for granted that it was going to work.

His right foot began shaking.

"*L'ap tremble,*" he croaked softly, pointing at his foot. ("It's shaking.")

It looked like clonus—a rapid, rhythmic oscillation of a part of the body that can occur with problems of the brain or spinal cord. It wasn't concerning, probably a residual effect of the tumor's long-term compression of his brain stem or from the surgeries.

I told him to shift his weight onto the trembling leg and push down a bit with his foot to make it go away. He did, and the shaking stopped. He smiled. I winked at him.

His mother and I approached him to support him, but he briskly shook his head once back and forth.

"Ale donc," his mother said, encouraging him. ("Go ahead, then.")

He stood for a few moments. Then, his arms still held out to the sides, he lifted his right foot slightly off the ground, stepped forward, and carefully set it down. After a pause, he slowly brought the other foot forward to meet it. Tentatively, he walked this way to cover the four steps from the mattress to the door, held on to the doorframe for balance while he carefully turned around, and then walked back to the mattress in the same way.

"L'ap mache pou kont li!" I said excitedly. ("He's walking on his own!")

His mother clapped, smiling broadly.

"Janel, ou mache byen!" I complimented him. ("Janel, you are walking well!")

He looked at me and then nodded his chin briskly upward.

"Mm!" his mother said proudly, closing her eyes and shaking her head. *"Apre Bondye se doktè!"* ("After God is the doctor!")

Janel's mom held his hand as he slowly squatted toward the mattress and then plopped the rest of the way down.

I explained to them that I thought Janel's dizziness was probably just a residual effect from his surgeries and possibly a slight side effect of his anti-seizure medication, or some combination of the two.

"But I don't think it's anything concerning," I said. "And it's great that he can walk a little."

"E li konn danse le m mete mizik," his mom added. ("And he sometimes dances if he hears music.")

Janel smiled and shook his head slowly, bashfully.

I told them I needed to return to the hospital. Janel's mom asked when I would be coming back. I told her I was leaving for Boston the next day but would come back on my next trip a few months later.

"*W prale lòt bò a demen si Bondye vle?*" she asked, pointing a hand outward and upward. ("You're going back to the other side tomorrow if God wants?")

"*Wi, demen,*" I said. ("Yes, tomorrow.")

"*Demen, si Bondye vle,*" she said, nodding. ("Tomorrow, if God wants.")

She walked with me down the three concrete stairs to the rocky path back to the main road. Some of her neighbors stared at us as we walked by, the strange sight of an elderly local lady and a young foreigner speaking to her in broken Creole.

When we reached the main dirt road to the hospital, she stopped.

"*M'ap kite ou la,*" she said. ("I'll let you go here.")

I told her I was happy to see her and Janel.

"*Salye tout moun pou mwen,*" she said, spreading her long arms wide. ("Say hi to everyone for me.") "*Remesye tout moun Boston—Madam Hermide, tout doktè!*" ("Thank everyone in Boston—Madame Hermide, all the doctors!")

I assured her I would.

We hugged, and I turned to walk to the hospital.

Janel wasn't doing great, but he was certainly doing better than before, I thought as I returned to HUM. Maybe we had helped him a little after all.

18

Pasteur came around quickly. The stutter and neglect went away after two days, and he was walking around after three. He was discharged from the hospital back to the room he shared with Dorotie in Joseph's apartment.

A week later, the pathology results came back: prolactinoma, a benign pituitary tumor. This was a huge relief. It meant that he didn't need chemotherapy or radiation.

Anne and I talked through the next steps. Pasteur required a medication to keep his tumor from growing back, and it wasn't available in Haiti. Despite the exorbitant prices that US pharmacies had quoted us for it, PIH staff found a way to get the medicine for a fraction of the cost from a medical distributor they worked with. But getting the pills delivered to Haiti would take time. We also thought Pasteur should stay in the US for a month to make sure there were no postoperative complications since it would be hard to get him back to Boston after he had returned to Haiti, especially if there was an emergency. Pasteur had told us he had a sister in Atlanta, so we thought maybe he and Dorotie would like to stay with her there just as Davidson and his father had stayed in Florida with their family while awaiting their final appointments.

I went to visit Pasteur and Dorotie at Joseph's to discuss everything with them. The window was open in their small room, looking out on a red brick wall a few feet away, the sounds of traffic floating in. Dorotie was sitting in a chair at the foot of the bed, typing on her phone. Pasteur was lying on the bed, wearing a white tank top and black shorts. The incision across his head was beginning to heal nicely, but his right eye remained closed even though the swelling around it had resolved. I examined the eye. The pupil didn't react and the eye could only move to the right but not up, down, or left—signs that one of the nerves to the eye had likely been injured during surgery.

"When will the eye open?" he asked me.

"If it was just injured during the surgery, it might open," I said. "But I have to be honest with you that it might stay closed if they had to sacrifice the nerve to get the whole tumor out. It's a small price to pay to cure you from the tumor, right?"

"I'm praying it will open," he replied.

"It may not, Pasteur," I told him bluntly. "We have to wait and see, but it may not. But I do have some good news."

Dorotie looked up from her phone.

"The tumor is benign. You don't need any radiation or chemotherapy!" I said.

They smiled at each other. *"Bondye gran!"* Dorotie said joyfully. ("God is great!")

"Louange à Dieu!" Pasteur intoned, raising his hands and looking upward. ("Praise to God!")

"When can we go home?" Dorotie asked. "We are trapped in this small apartment." She explained that Joseph spent a lot of time outside the apartment, and they weren't comfortable going out on their own.

"We think you should stay in the US for another month to make sure everything goes okay," I began, "but I have an idea I think you will like. What if we fly you to Atlanta to stay with your sister?" I smiled at them expectantly.

"Oh no! Atlanta two lwen!" Pasteur said. ("Atlanta is too far away!")

"Wi, li two lwen!" Dorotie concurred. ("Yes, it's too far!")

My smile faded as I cocked my head to the side, confused. I had thought they would love the idea. Before I had a chance to explain that we would pay for their flights in case that was a concern, Pasteur asked, *"Poukisa pa New York?"* ("Why not New York?")

"Oh, do you know people in New York?" I asked, surprised.

"New York, New Jersey," Pasteur said with casual confidence, waving one hand lazily back and forth. "We know lots of people there."

"Okay," I said, laughing, "we can arrange that."

"My brother can come pick us up on Thursday and drive us back to his house in New York, no problem," Pasteur said.

I laughed again. "Okay, it sounds like you have it all figured out, then."

When I later told Anne about this, she told me she'd seen the "family members living in the US who magically appear" story countless times with patients who came to the US from Haiti for surgery. She wondered if patients didn't disclose it out of fear it could jeopardize their medical visa application.

"Could this surgery have been done in Haiti?" Dorotie asked me.

"Well, technically the surgeon could have gone to Haiti and tried to do the surgery," I said, "but it's such a big operation requiring very careful monitoring, so we didn't think it was safe."

"Can anyone in Haiti do this surgery?" Pasteur asked.

"I don't think so," I said. "It requires a real expert like Dr. Ian Dunn—he is specialized in brain tumor surgery and does more than two hundred brain tumor surgeries each year!"

"This is God's work that you got us here!" Pasteur exclaimed, enunciating each word. "No Haitian could get me here because they don't speak English!" His voice began taking on a preacher's prosody, each sentence infused with more passion and intensity than the last. "And you speak English, and so God acted through you. He acted through you to get me this care! To get me to Boston!! *Bondye ap pran note!! Glwa a Dye!!!*" ("God is noticing!! Glory to God!!!")

"Amen!!!"

"Amen," Dorotie said.

I was leaving on vacation the next week with Nina and assured

Pasteur and Dorotie that Anne would help them get to New York and then back to Boston for his follow-up appointments. I felt bad to be leaving, but between work in the hospital, a five-week neurology course I had just finished teaching at the medical school, and the parallel full-time job of coordinating Pasteur's care—all things I loved doing, but a tiring combination nonetheless—I was glad to get away to relax a little, and the timing turned out to be perfect since Pasteur seemed to have sailed smoothly through his surgery.

They wished me a good trip.

As I left, I tried out a joke I'd been saving for the right moment. I had noticed Pasteur and Dorotie's affectionate nicknames for each other. So on my way out, I said, *"Si ou DoDo e ou JeanJean, ou ka rele'm 'RonRon'!"* ("If you go by DoDo and you go by JeanJean, then you can call me 'RonRon'!")

They burst into laughter. *"Dako, Doktè RonRon!"* Pasteur said, continuing to laugh as I left. ("Okay, Doctor RonRon!")

"Wi, Doktè Ti'RonRon!" laughed Dorotie. ("Yes, Doctor Little RonRon!")

As they closed the door, I heard them still laughing and saying *"Doktè RonRon."* I smiled. I remembered the uncomfortable feeling I'd had leaving on my honeymoon when Janel hadn't even woken up from his first surgery. Little did I know then that he had four more in his future. This time, I left for vacation feeling all was well.

———

Nina and I had decided to spend our vacation in Iceland, driving around the country in a campervan—a van with a small foldout bed and kitchen in the back. Driving in Iceland is spectacular, with extraordinary landscapes at every turn. But it's also filled with various obstacles: dense fog, one-lane bridges and tunnels requiring careful choreography with oncoming traffic, winding fjord roads with steep drop-offs to the ocean below, and sheep. Lots of sheep.

Iceland has more sheep than people. Sheep often meander onto the road unexpectedly, appearing out of nowhere, and are a major cause of car accidents. We were somewhere between the unpronounceable small villages of Höfn and Seydisfjördur in southeast Iceland when we saw several cars stopped ahead on the road. We slowed to a halt.

"Sheep crossing?" I joked to Nina. A few people were standing outside their cars in front of us looking down the steep grassy slope to the left of the road. Following their gaze into the ravine, I saw a jeep at the bottom with two parallel swerving lines of torn-up grass behind it.

"Oh no, they must have run off the road," Nina said.

Looking into the distance, I could make out a few people standing outside the jeep. There was a large white shape in front of them. Was it a sheep? Did they hit a sheep and swerve off the road? I got out of our van to get a better look.

I squinted into the sun. They weren't standing around a sheep—they were standing around a person lying on the ground. My body lurched into medical emergency fight-or-flight mode.

"Maybe I should go down there?" I asked Nina through the van window. "Just to see if they need a doctor?"

Nina looked at me, concerned. "Are you sure?"

I hesitated. "Okay, I'm going to head down there," I said, convincing myself. I started jogging across the road from where we had pulled over.

"Be careful!" Nina shouted after me from the van.

I half ran, half slid down the slope, amazed that the jeep hadn't flipped over on the way down.

As I approached, it became clear that the white shape was the glistening torso and abdomen of an obese old man lying in the grass a few feet from the skid marks that led to the jeep. A younger man was performing vigorous, rhythmic chest compressions with his hands one on top of the other causing the protuberant belly of the man on the ground to ripple wildly. Another young man was performing mouth-to-mouth breathing. An older woman and a young man stood off to the side, watching anxiously.

Seeing the attempted resuscitation in action, my adrenaline began pumping even harder. Neurologists fortunately don't participate in too many code blue situations. I tried to remember the last time I had coded someone. It had probably been years ago when I was an intern. I suddenly had a flashback of my senior resident yelling at me that my chest compressions were not deep and strong enough. She had swapped me out to do a less physical task.

"I'm a doctor," I said as I nervously walked toward them. "Can I help?"

The two men looked up at me without breaking the rhythm of their resuscitation. "I'm a nurse," the man thumping the patient's chest said in accented English, breathing heavily. "And he's a doctor," he added, nodding his head toward the other man performing mouth-to-mouth breathing.

"Do you need an extra set of hands?" I asked.

"No," the mouth-to-mouth breather said between breaths, "we're just trying to get some air into this guy!"

They continued their resuscitation attempt.

I lingered for a moment. Then, seeing as they didn't seem to think I could help, I scampered back up the grassy hill to our campervan.

Nina rolled down the driver's side window. "What's going on?" she asked.

"They were coding him," I said to her through the window, slightly out of breath from both the run up the hill and my adrenaline-fueled response to the emergency before I saw others were taking care of it. "They said they didn't need me." I caught my breath. "I wonder if he had a heart attack and skidded off the road and someone else in the car grabbed the wheel so they didn't flip over. It didn't look like there had been an accident since nobody else was hurt."

"I hope he'll be okay," Nina said, starting the car. I got into the passenger's seat, closed my eyes, and took a deep breath. My heart was still galloping in my chest, my pulse pounding in my ears.

We pulled slowly around the stopped cars and regained our pace on the ring road that circumnavigates the country.

"You okay?" Nina asked.

"Yeah," I said. "The people trying to revive him said they were a doctor and a nurse. I wonder if they were friends or family members in the car with him who happened to be medical people or some type of emergency first responders who got there really quickly."

"Oh wow," Nina said.

"Can you believe it?" I asked. "Less than three hundred thousand people live in Iceland and we are literally in the middle of nowhere here, but there was a doctor and a nurse down there!"

We drove on in silence through the verdant mountainous landscape, the grass on the hills so green it looked neon in the midday sun, the fluffy clouds on the horizon so perfectly spaced that they appeared painted onto the scene.

I imagined a family in Haiti carrying a body up a hill, two people holding the arms, two holding the legs. Once they got to the road, they'd prop the body onto the back of a hired motorcycle to get to the nearest hospital, which could be hours away. By the time they made it to the hospital, the patient would surely be what we call DOA: dead on arrival. There are more than ten million people in Haiti, but what would have been the chances of having one—let alone two—medical personnel at the site of a medical emergency so quickly, either by chance or by design? And here I was, just an extra doctor that nobody even needed!

If your eyes are open, I thought, reminders of inequity are everywhere.

I closed my eyes and tried to convince myself it was okay to be on vacation.

When I got back from Iceland, I called Pasteur in New York to check in with him. He and Dorotie were doing well, enjoying being surrounded by his family. I heard his nephews and nieces laughing and playing in the background. He put them on the phone so they could practice their English with me, and then he put his brother on the phone to show him *"Doktè mwen ka pale Kreyol!"* ("My doctor can speak Creole!")

When Pasteur's brother brought him and Dorotie back to Boston for a day of final appointments before they returned to Haiti, I met them in the lobby at Brigham. Pasteur was wearing a black New York Yankees hat his brother had bought him. Unfortunately, his right eyelid was still closed.

"W moun New York kounyea?" I asked him, smiling as we shook hands. ("You a New York guy now?")

"No, mwen moun Boston!" he exclaimed, smiling back. *"Paske se nan Boston Bondye te swenye'm!"* ("No, I'm a Boston guy! Because it's in Boston that God cured me!")

Pasteur had his last appointments at Brigham and gave all of the doctors, nurses, and staff his thanks and blessings. As we said our goodbyes, Pasteur gave me two envelopes, one for me and one for Anne.

"Mesi pou tou bagay ou te fè pou mwen," he said, smiling softly. ("Thank you for everything you did for me.")

I choked up. "Thanks for your patience and courage. I'm sorry it took us so long, but I'm so glad it all finally worked out."

"Gras a Dye!" he said, pointing his index finger upward. ("Thanks to God!") *"E apre Bondye se doktè!"* he added, smiling. ("And after God is the doctor!")

"No, no," I laughed.

"DoDo and I will come visit you in Mirebalais when you come to HUM," he said.

"Great, and you contact me on WhatsApp if there are any problems or questions," I said.

We hugged.

He and Dorotie got into his brother's car and they drove off, waving to me as they passed. I smiled and waved until I lost sight of their car.

When I got home that night and unpacked my workbag, I saw the envelope from Pasteur mixed in with some papers and opened it.

Inside was a Hallmark greeting card on which Pasteur had written in perfect cursive:

> *We make a living by what we get, but we make a life by what we give. After God, you Doctors give me life. Words can't express how grateful and thankful I am for all your support. From the bottom of my heart in just two words . . . Thank you.*
>
> *Gratefully, Jean-Rémy*

19

Squinting into the blazing midday Haitian sun, I saw Michelle standing next to a white jeep near the entrance to HUM. She waved me over. Just as I was about to reach her, the passenger door of the jeep opened, and out stepped Paul Farmer. As I approached to greet them, Paul was telling Michelle that he had arrived a little early for a meeting he had later in the afternoon.

"Do you want to go see a patient in the community?" Michelle asked him.

"Always up for a home visit," he said. He pulled a wide-brimmed straw hat from his backpack and put it on. "Otherwise this cracker will get sunburned!" he said, smirking.

"Let's take him to meet Janel," Michelle said, winking at me as Paul put his hat on. I had told Michelle about my disappointing debate with Paul a few months prior when I had tried unsuccessfully to engage him to help us advocate for bringing patients from Haiti to Boston for neurosurgery. I suspected she was hoping that visiting Janel—and Paul's inevitable connection with him and his story—would inspire him to support us in our efforts to care for more brain tumor patients in Boston, theoretical debates aside.

Paul often bonded closely with patients. During a previous visit to HUM, he was invited to give a lecture to the hospital staff. Paul asked the staff to choose a patient at HUM for him to examine and discuss at the lecture. They took him to meet a twelve-year-old boy in the intensive care unit who had become completely paralyzed from Guillain-Barré syndrome, most likely due to Zika infection. Even the boy's respiratory muscles had become paralyzed, requiring a ventilator to breathe for him through a tracheostomy, a hole cut in his throat. The boy was just beginning to recover, starting to breath on his own, speak, and move his limbs a little. He was an HUM success story—he would have died without the support of the ventilator, suffocating to death.

Paul sat on the boy's hospital bed and interviewed him about his illness. Paul's bedside manner was incredible, his Creole fluent. He was able to elicit details of the patient's history that had eluded us. He bonded with the boy, bought him a cell phone so they could keep in touch, and visited him on subsequent trips. In his lecture, Paul held the boy's story up as an example of why we couldn't wait until primary care was perfected to begin providing advanced medical treatment like intensive care in places like rural Haiti.

We waited for a break in the motorcycle traffic to cross the street in front of the hospital, then set off on the chalky, rocky, trash-lined path that led into the community. A large truck approached behind us, taking up the entire dirt road. We stepped to the side and were enveloped in a hot cloud of road dust and diesel fumes. As we turned onto the small path to Janel's house, a chicken scuttled by with chirping yellow chicks in tow. A bare-bummed young boy ran past wearing only a T-shirt, trailing a small pink-striped plastic bag attached to a short string in the air behind him—flying a makeshift kite.

I summarized Janel's story for Paul along the way. The huge tumor that had left Janel barely able to move or speak. The amazing team that had rallied around him at Brigham. The rarity of the tumor, a type that none of us had ever heard of, requiring several surgeries, radiation, and chemotherapy. PIH's efforts to relocate Janel and his mom closer to the hospital and provide them with monthly support for food. I admitted that he hadn't done as well as we'd hoped, but he could walk a few steps and say a few words, which he couldn't do before surgery.

We ascended the three concrete steps to their house.

"What was the name of that tumor again?" Paul asked as we stood in front of their wooden door.

"PPTID—pineal parenchymal tumor of intermediate differentiation." I said.

He jotted it down in a small pocket notebook. "Never heard of that one," he said. "I'll have to read up on it."

We knocked. Janel's mom opened the door slightly to peek out, smiled broadly, and then opened the door wide. "Oo-eee, Dok!" she shouted joyfully. "Oo-eee, Doktè Michelle! Doktè Aaron! Oo-eee!" she nearly sang as she kissed us on each cheek. We introduced Doktè Paul, and she invited us in.

Janel was sitting on his mattress in the middle of the floor. His mom unstacked her three white plastic lawn chairs, placing them in a semicircle around the front of the mattress. She motioned excitedly for us to sit, then sat in the corner behind us on a small wood-and-wicker stool just a few inches off the ground. Janel reached forward to greet each of us with a handshake, a smile, and a "Kouman ou ye, Dok?" ("How are you, Doc?")

Michelle and I looked at each other, eyebrows raised in disbelief. "Wow!" she said. "He looks amazing!"

"So much better," I concurred, surprised at how much more engaged he appeared. "Kouman ou ye?" I asked Janel as we sat down. ("How are you?")

"Oooo, Dok," he said in his high-pitched, scratchy voice, slapping the back of one hand into the palm of the other. "M gen gwo doulè, wi!" ("I've got a lot of pain!")

"He's had headaches since his surgeries," I told Paul. "That's no surprise after all he's been through, but he looks so much better than when we last saw him a few months ago—more alert, attentive, and quick in his responses. To be honest, I can't believe it.

"W gen toujou tèt fè mal, Janel, pa vre?" I asked. ("You still get headaches, Janel, isn't that right?") I was eager to know how he was doing but also realized a bit sheepishly that I was trying to impress Paul with my Creole.

"*Pa nan tèt, no, Dok!*" Janel replied emphatically, shaking his head with his eyes closed and waving one hand adamantly back and forth. "*Nan kè!*" ("Not in my head, no, Doc! In my heart!")

I squinted at Michelle and cocked my head to the side, confused.

Janel continued. "*M gen gwo doulè nan kè a paske m vle tounen lekòl!*" ("I have this big pain in my heart because I want to go back to school!")

Paul looked sharply at me. "Haven't you read any of my books?" he asked sternly, then flashed a grin. "The most important part of the medical history is the social history. His pain is not from his surgery, it's due to social factors. Come on, Social Medicine 101."

"Well, this is the first time he's mentioned anything about school," I said, caught off guard and embarrassed. "Last time we saw him . . ." I trailed off. "Last time we saw him he could . . . he could just barely speak, so this is . . . well . . . this is . . . a huge change."

Paul talked a bit with Janel about going back to school. He threw in Creole slang and jokes that made Janel laugh.

Then Janel launched into a long monologue. I was amazed at how fluid and animated his speech was but couldn't understand much of it since my Creole was still limited. "What's he saying?" I asked Michelle discreetly.

"Wow," she said quietly, keeping her gaze focused on Janel. "He's saying that if he can't go to school, he's afraid he won't be able to take care of his mom in the future. And he's throwing in all kinds of proverbs. Deep stuff."

Unable to follow the Creole, I just sat back and took it all in. Paul and Janel chatted. Michelle listened, nodding slowly, smiling softly, her eyes slightly narrowed. She looked moved. Janel's mother beamed from her wood-and-wicker stool. Her son was well, her new home filled with guests. The translucent pink curtains flapped gently in a light breeze, letting varying amounts of sunlight into the dim house as they billowed slowly toward and away from the window openings.

I turned my attention to Paul Farmer. He was leaning toward Janel, listening intently. His posture appeared to me simultaneously that of a compassionate physician and an attuned anthropologist, the complementary roles that defined his career. I imagined his trip to HUM would involve high-level strategic meetings with local PIH/ZL leadership and government ministers about protocols, procedures, and budgets. Perhaps he'd lecture on a topic in infectious diseases to the HUM internal medicine residents. Maybe he'd give a tour to visiting donors in which he would narrate the history of Haiti and PIH/ZL, infused with quotations from sociology and philosophy. But before all that, he was making a house call, seeing a patient.

The scene felt to me like it could be right out of the book *Mountains Beyond Mountains: The Quest of Dr. Paul Farmer, A Man Who Would Cure the World* by Tracy Kidder. Except, I realized, I was in the scene.

How long had it been since I had read *Mountains Beyond Mountains*? I calculated back—almost exactly eight years. I could remember that moment clearly. Disillusioned with the drudgery of medical school, I had decided to take a leave of absence to pursue my first love: music. I found my way into a PhD program in musicology and was elated with my decision to take the road less traveled. I was so much happier than I had been when I was standing on endless hospital rounds in my short white coat and poring over board-review books in the medical school library stacks. Instead, I was spending my days playing the piano, taking courses in music theory and history, and doing research on music and the brain. With much more free time than I'd had as a medical student, I swam, I took tai chi and yoga classes, and I went on meditation retreats.

After about five years away from medical school, I was pretty sure I wasn't going to go back. I had come to enjoy the freedom and relaxed pace of life in the academic humanities and was imagining myself as a music professor in a small liberal arts college after I finished my PhD. I felt that by leaving medicine I had dodged a bullet, escaping a lifetime of working too much and too hard.

Then, within a one-week period, I heard both Bill Clinton and Bill Gates lecture about the work their foundations were doing. They spoke about poverty and inequity, about HIV, tuberculosis, and malaria, about tsunami and earthquake relief. Clinton described how he was struck by how the human genome project demonstrated that humans are 99.9 percent similar and only 0.1 percent different and how this underscored what he felt Nelson Mandela, Mother Teresa, and Martin Luther King had embodied: "What we have in common is more important than what divides us." Clinton proclaimed that "ordinary people have more power to do public good than ever before" and implored us to "spend as much of your time and your heart and your spirit as you possibly can thinking about the other 99.9 percent."

Gates said he believed that our generation had access to technology and awareness of global inequity that his generation did not. "And with that awareness," he said, "you likely also have an informed conscience that will torment you if you abandon these people whose lives you could change with very little effort. You have more than we had; you must start sooner, and carry on longer. Knowing what you know, how could you not? And I hope you will . . . thirty years from now . . . reflect on what you have done with your talent and your energy. I hope you will judge yourselves not on your professional accomplishments alone, but also on how well you have addressed the world's deepest inequities . . . on how well you treated people a world away who have nothing in common with you but their humanity."

Gates's and Clinton's words struck a deep chord in me. The underground piano practice room where I spent most of my waking hours suddenly felt small. All that yoga and meditation had done its work on my mind: a life of selfless service was calling. I started to feel like maybe I should go back to medical school after all.

But it was reading *Mountains Beyond Mountains* around that time that definitively spun my inner compass back toward medicine after years of trying to escape it. There was so much suffering and inequity in the world, and I was just one year away from a medical degree that might allow me to try to help do something about it, however small. I set my sights on working with PIH someday.

In the year before I went back to medical school, I began auditing classes in public health and medical anthropology while I finished writing my musicology dissertation. I snuck away for one month to Guatemala to learn Spanish and volunteer in a free clinic and worked with a US-based neurologist who was setting up an epilepsy program in the Ecuadorian Amazon. After what had been a prolonged period of waffling between whether I should become a musician or a doctor, everything took on a certain momentum, each year flying by faster than the last—the final year of medical school, internship, neurology residency.

And suddenly here I was, in the place where PIH had begun, sitting with Paul Farmer, "a man who would cure the world." A man who had sat here thirty years ago doing exactly what he was doing now, and what he taught us to do: listen to the poor, accompany them, fight for them. A man who helped galvanize a generation and inspire a movement that I was swept up in, Michelle was swept up in, Janel and his tumor and his mother and their house were swept up in. Sitting there, I briefly had the rare experience of being fully in the moment, a moment that felt like it was the culmination of all the moments leading up to it, as though everything had turned out just as it was meant to and I had come full circle.

"*M ka tounen pi ta ak kek zanmi'm?*" Paul asked Janel. ("Can I come back later with some friends?")

"*Pa gen pwoblem, Dok!*" Janel agreed. ("No problem, Doc!")

I imagined that Paul wanted to introduce Janel to some donors as a PIH success story—a triumph against the impossible.

We said our goodbyes and thank-yous to Janel and his mom and headed back to the hospital.

"We've got to get this boy back to school!" Paul said as we walked on the dirt path back to HUM. "Come on, haven't you read any of my books?" he teased, cracking a smile.

"From *AIDS and Accusation* to *Reimagining Global Health*," I replied, smiling back proudly. It was true.

He laughed. "Some of them are real sleepers, I admit."

A motorcycle noisily swerved around us on the dirt road. Several scrawny barking dogs chased after it, then gave up and lay down in the shade of a banana tree on the side of the road.

"There are going to be more brain tumor patients here we will want to try to get to Brigham," I said, unable to resist the urge to make something of the moment.

"Send me a list of all the people at Brigham who helped Janel," Paul replied. "Let me write them an email thanking them for all they did for him. It's really incredible."

Michelle winked at me from behind Paul.

"That would be great," I said. "Thank you."

"Ian Dunn is a magician," Paul said. "He has saved more than one of my patients, but Janel takes the cake. His case wouldn't have gone well in Haiti, but there will be easier ones that will. Tell Ian he has a standing invitation from me to come down here."

"I'll let him know," I replied.

We got back to the hospital and went our separate ways.

When I went back to visit Janel later on during that trip, he was proudly sporting a brand-new pair of Ray-Ban sunglasses, a gift from *Doktè Paul*. The glasses probably cost more than Janel and his mother's monthly allowance, I thought cynically. But to Janel they were a treasure. I remembered how Paul had justified his plan for building botanical gardens at HUM when we looked at him skeptically: the work should be beautiful, not just functional. Seeing Janel smile at me in his hip new shades, I realized Paul was making another teaching point.

20

I was tracking the path of Hurricane Irma, which looked like it was headed straight for Haiti. I received alerts in Boston that PIH was considering evacuating visiting staff, including one of my colleagues I had recruited to teach in our neurology training program. As the meteorological models updated day by day, it looked like Irma was going to mostly spare Haiti but could still graze the northern tip of the island. I zoomed in on the map to see what area was in its path: Port-de-Paix, where Enel and Davidson lived. I sent Enel a message through WhatsApp to say I hoped they would be okay in spite of the storm.

> Me: Is it raining a lot there?

> Enel: Lots of strong wind and rain this morning.

> Me: I hope your house will be OK.

> Enel: Yes, we are praying to God that this storm won't touch our house, thank you.

Then his status was "Offline." I sent him a message and it didn't go through.

I tried again the next morning, but he was still offline.

I began to worry. I saw a news story that lamented there was no hurricane notification system in this part of Haiti, and even if there had been, there were no evacuation shelters for residents to take shelter in. I heard rumors that the Haitian government had allotted only five thousand dollars to hurricane relief.

I had the morbid thought of what a truly tragic twist it would be if Davidson had made it all the way to Boston for a complex neurosurgery and back to Haiti healthy, only to die in a natural disaster. Or rather an *un*natural disaster, as Paul Farmer would call it, since natural disasters cause greater damage and loss of life in poor regions, where there are limited resources for preparation and recovery.

Finally, later the next day, Enel replied:

> We are OK, the storm didn't touch my house. God protected me.

21

As I approached Janel's house, his mom came from around the back wearing a tight black cap that held her short gray braids away from her forehead, a black T-shirt with a gray peace sign and PEACE in big white block letters across it, and a black skirt. She saw me, smiled broadly, and came to greet me.

She led me up the steps to where Janel was sitting outside on the porch in a white plastic lawn chair eating red beans and rice out of a metal bowl. He was wearing a torn brown tank top and black gym shorts—and his Ray-Ban sunglasses from Paul Farmer.

Janel put his fork and bowl down in his lap and reached out his hand.

"Bonjou, Janel!" I said, shaking his hand. ("Hi, Janel!")

Janel gripped my hand in a tight handshake, then shifted his grip so we had our thumbs linked and held each other's wrists, then shifted back to a normal handshake, then quickly back again to the thumb grip. Then he pulled his hand away, made a fist, and tapped his chest with it.

"Wow!" I laughed.

He smiled broadly. *"Respè,"* he said, nodding coolly. ("Respect.")

His mother brought another white plastic lawn chair out from the house for me, and I sat down. She squatted across from us on the porch, pulling the back of her skirt up through her legs. Next to her, an adorable toddler in a pink tank top was sitting bare-bummed on the concrete floor, her baby-fat legs splayed out to her sides, her hair in countless tiny braids, her little ears adorned with miniature gold hoop earrings. She was playing with a green bottle cap and an empty plastic soda bottle. Beside her, a chicken was frantically trying to figure out why it couldn't walk more than two steps from the wood-and-wicker stool to which one of its clawed yellow feet was tied with twine. The chicken occasionally flapped its wings and squawked in frustration, and the infant cooed with delight and flapped her hands in response.

I asked Janel's mother if the chicken was hers. She proudly said yes, explaining that Janel's father had bought it for them.

I had never met Janel's father. Martineau had seen him only once over the years.

"*Janel, kouman rele poule a?*" I asked him. ("Janel, what's the chicken's name?")

"*Dyekibay,*" he said, grinning broadly.

I didn't understand. "*Kouman?*" I asked him. ("What?")

He kept smiling. "*Dyekibay!*" he said and laughed. His mother laughed too.

"*Dyekibay?*" I asked, still confused.

He leaned slightly forward toward me, nodding slowly, waiting for me to get it.

I shook my head.

"Ah, *Dye-ki-bay,*" I finally said, separating it into its component words: *Dye* (God), *ki* (who), *bay* (gives).

He gave a quick nod up of his chin, clapped, and then reached his hand out for another elaborate handshake.

"*W pral manje'l, Janel?*" I asked him. ("Are you going to eat it, Janel?")

"*No, se Bondye ki pral manje'l!*" he declared happily. ("No, God is going to eat it!")

His mother burst out laughing. "*Li ba'y blag tout jounen!*" she said, clapping contentedly. ("He tells jokes all day!")

I was amazed to see Janel sitting on his porch cracking jokes and making secret handshakes when just a few months prior he had been bedbound and mute with a fixed, wide-eyed stare—and a few months before that, comatose. I felt a strange mixture of joy at how well things had turned out for him and regret over all of the times I had nearly given up hope that any good would come from having tried to help him without really knowing how.

"Janel, Bondye pa ka manje poule a," I said, laughing and trying to participate in his joke. ("Janel, God can't eat that chicken.")

"Men se Bondye ki ba'm fòs pou manje'l!" he said, without missing a beat, and broke into his full-on Cheshire-cat smile. ("But it is God who will give me the strength to eat it!")

Now we all laughed.

His mom explained that they hoped the chicken would have chicks, which they would sell to help pay for Janel to go back to school. She said their neighbor was sewing a school uniform for him. Hearing reference to his work, the neighbor came out onto his porch, a muscular, shirtless young man who looked to be in his early twenties. He told me he hadn't been paid yet for the uniform and asked when someone from the hospital would be bringing him his money. I told him I would ask Martineau. Then he showed me a keloid—a raised, prominent scar—on his upper arm. He wanted to know if I could get it fixed for him in the US. While I tried to explain that I didn't know much about keloids but that I didn't think so, an older thin man with a short white beard emerged from the door, his dark eyes clouded by milky cataracts.

"E mwen menm," he said, *"w ka ede'm ak kò mwen, Dok?"* ("And what about me, can you help me with my body, Doc?")

I asked him what was wrong and couldn't understand much of what he said in response, but he kept pointing to his stomach. I encouraged him to go to HUM to get evaluated by a doctor. I tried to explain that I was a *newolog* (neurologist)—a *doktè tèt* (head doctor)—and that I didn't know much about problems of the skin or abdomen. Disappointed, they went back inside.

Since Janel was so interactive now, I wanted to ask him some of the questions I'd always wondered about. Maybe I could finally begin to understand that period when his behavior had been so confusing to us.

I asked him if he had been scared to come to Boston.

He shook his head briskly no, pointed one finger upward, grinned, and then shimmied both hands in front of him in a gesture I'd seen Pasteur make a number of times when saying *"Louange à Dieu"* ("Praise to God").

I asked him if he had been scared to have surgery.

He repeated the same series of gestures.

I asked his mom if she had been scared when Janel left for Boston. She reached her long, thin arms up to the clear blue cloudless sky and looked up as if to receive the rains from heaven.

"Li te nan men Bondye!" she exclaimed, smiling. *"E apre sa nan men doktè. Nou te pa pè, no!"* ("He was in the hands of God! And after that in the hands of the doctors. We weren't scared, no!")

22

I looked up from my laptop. Thick clouds had obscured the sunset, bathing the evening sky in a strange orange-pink-gray hue. I was sitting on the balcony of the HUM staff house because it was just too hot and stuffy in my room and it was a few degrees cooler outside. Beyond the barbed-wire-topped wall surrounding the house, across a small dirt road, a stray dog and a goat ambled in the yard outside a tin-roofed shack. A young boy wearing an orange tank top and gray underwear joyfully brandished a stick and banged it against the broad trunk of a mango tree.

My bags were all packed to head home to Boston the next morning.

I'm always sad to leave Haiti, and I wish I had more time there. But it had been a rough trip, and at one point I had caught myself counting the remaining days. The temperature was hotter than I'd ever experienced in Haiti—even my Haitian colleagues were complaining about the heat. The electricity was unpredictable, leaving several nights without lights or fans. I had gotten some very itchy rash on my legs either from bug bites, heat, or who knows what. One morning after a broiling, fan-less night, we awoke to find there was no water—we went off to work dirty and dehydrated from a midsummer night's sweat. And although I felt I should have been above complaining about it, the hospital internet was at its most temperamental, making it hard to keep up with work and life back in Boston.

When the last day of a trip to Haiti arrives, I always feel guilty and embarrassed for having had any adverse reactions during my time there.

My minor inconveniences could hardly be called suffering compared to what our patients experience. Most of them have never had running water or electricity at home to lose.

I was concerned that on this particular trip my physical discomfort might have interfered with my ability to do my work as well as I aspired to. I worried I hadn't been persistent enough to make sure I truly understood what was said by our neurology trainees and their patients in each encounter. I was afraid I had let things slide so the day wouldn't drag on too late, overly influenced by my not-so-subconscious eagerness to get through our work, go back to the staff house, peel off my sweaty work clothes, take a cold shower (if there was water), and put my heat-swollen feet up.

I wondered what it would be like to live in Haiti, truly settling in for the long haul of a year or two or more. Maybe it would feel easier when it wasn't a circumscribed two-week period during which minor discomforts get magnified because they aren't the norm. Maybe I would adjust to the struggle of life in Haiti. Maybe someday, I told myself. As the sun set on this trip, I promised myself I would try harder to be more mindful the next time I was here to make the most of my brief visits.

But the trip had its high points too. Janel looked so much better than we could have ever imagined. François was about to become the first graduate of our two-year neurology training program. He and I had nostalgically reminisced about what a journey it had been for both of us. We had counted that this was my eleventh or twelfth trip to Haiti in the preceding two years. I had lost count, but my passport was so filled with Haiti customs stamps that I needed a new one.

François had worked and studied incredibly hard, developing into a brilliant neurologist and teacher. He diagnosed Haiti's first cases of Guillain-Barré syndrome due to Zika infection. He published a report on this, which led to a scholarship to the American Academy of Neurology annual meeting in Boston, where he gave a lecture presenting

his work. We were told by one of the scholarship committee members
that François was the first Haitian national to have ever attended the
conference. As our neurology program's pioneer trainee, François had
done so phenomenally well that HUM was planning to hire him with
the goal of having him eventually take over the leadership of the program. Maybe HUM would have a self-sustaining locally run neurology
program even sooner than we had hoped.

"Ce doit être la grande providence qui m'a amené ici à Mirebalais,"
Dr. François said to me. ("It must have been divine providence that
brought me here to Mirebalais.")

In addition to being a rigorous clinician and scientist, François is
also deeply religious. He told me that he had bought a plot of land in
Mirebalais not far from HUM years before there was even a plan to
build a hospital in the town, let alone a major teaching hospital. Tired
of city life in Port-au-Prince, he set up the land to farm corn and
mangoes, and was even thinking of leaving medicine entirely to work
the land. With the construction of HUM, François's land increased in
value, so he held on to it and kept working in his government hospital post in Port-au-Prince. One day a colleague there showed him a
newspaper clipping announcing a neurology residency run by a faculty member from Harvard. The location was Mirebalais. François had
always wanted to advance his training by studying a specialty, but there
had never been an opportunity in Haiti. And now there was one right
next to the land he had purchased many years earlier.

"I know you are not religious, Dr. Aaron," he said, "but how do
you explain the coincidences—the land, the hospital, the neurology
program—that brought us both here to this small town of Mirebalais?
How do you explain it if not divine providence?"

François had asked me, based on my name, if I was Jewish. When
I told him that my family was Jewish but I wasn't practicing any religion, he was taken aback. I laughed and told him that my religion was
neurology: I reread its texts daily, it gives me a framework for thinking

through difficult problems, and it provides me with the tools to work in the service of others—didn't that make it a religion?

He was not amused. "No!" he exclaimed. "Neurology is not a religion! Look, the Jews are a great people. With all this work you do for the poor in our country, if you would just listen to your great-great-great-great grandfather Abraham and pray to the God of your ancestors, you would become a saint!"

I laughed. "I'm content to be a neurologist," I told him.

He shook his head and laughed too.

Yes, these trips had their joys as well as their difficulties, I thought as I typed up some notes on the progress of the neurology training program at the two-year mark.

I looked down from the balcony at the boy across the road, still pants-less, still gleefully hitting the mango tree with his stick as night fell, the smoky smell of cooking fires beginning to fill the air. And here I was, slathered in insect repellent, typing on my laptop, a generator-powered electric fan blowing on my back, a packet of organic low-sodium ramen soup cooking on the gas-powered stove inside.

How did I end up up here and the boy down there? If I had begun down there, would I have had the drive and persistence of Martineau to rise out of poverty and become a doctor, and the humility to return to serve the poor if I had succeeded? Would I have died a stupid death from tuberculosis, malaria, or malnutrition before I even made it to school? Or would I have made it to early adulthood only to die from a condition that could have been treated a short flight away, like Francky? Would people sit on the balcony looking down at me, shaking their heads at how unlucky I was to have been born in Haiti?

Paul Farmer would say it's not about being unlucky to have been born in one place and lucky to have been born in another. He would explain that it has nothing to do with luck at all but rather with the forces of history, economics, and politics that create and continue to deepen such inequities.

And to those who shrug and talk about bad luck, he would probably retort with one of his most famous quotations: "The idea that some lives matter less is the root of all that's wrong with the world."

If that idea is the root of all that is wrong in the world, then perhaps the Haitian proverb *Tout moun se moun*—Every person is a person—could be the root of all that is good. If we began by assuming we are all equal, we would see no choice but to work toward closing the gaps in equity where they gape. The principle is simple, but the practice can be complex, as the stories told in this book have taught me. But we have to do whatever it takes. Anything less would be, to quote Paul again, "a failure of imagination."

Pasteur is back preaching in Gonaïves. I see him and Dorotie when I'm in Mirebalais and they come to pick up his medications at HUM. His right eye never opened, but the scar on his scalp is barely visible—it didn't form a keloid as he had worried about.

Davidson continues with school in Port-de-Paix. He actively plays sports. He and his dad live too far from Mirebalais to visit when I'm in Haiti, but his dad and I exchange texts from time to time. When I ask how he is, he often replies: *"Nou anfom ak sekou Jezi"* ("We are fine with the protection of Jesus"). He wrote to me recently that Davidson wants to be a doctor when he grows up.

We did try to get Janel back to school. But after going for a few days, he appeared depressed and didn't return. We never fully understood what happened, and he gradually returned to his jokes and elaborate handshakes. Our suspicion was that unfortunately he may have overestimated himself, and we may have overestimated him. But nearly four years after his surgeries, *li la*—he's here. Maybe he wasn't quite the big save we had hoped for. But he was the big save his mom had hoped for.

PIH continues to work toward developing sustainable healthcare systems for the poorest patients in the most destitute regions of the world. They're making incredible progress. But not fast enough for the Janels, the Davidsons, and the Pasteurs who need the future—the present that the rest of us take for granted—to be now. Although we somehow found a way to bring these patients to modern medicine, I don't deny that our critics are right: what we did isn't cost-effective and it's not sustainable.

But neither is the alternative.

Epilogue

Martineau sat across from me at my kitchen table in Boston. Over the last several years, he had taken the three eight-hour examinations necessary to apply for residency training in the US and aced them. He decided to apply in neurology and was offered a position in Boston, overcoming the significant hurdles for international physicians applying into the US system. We talked about what lay ahead for him in his training, and the conversation eventually turned to reminiscing about Janel. He filled in aspects of Janel's story in Haiti—and his own—that I hadn't known about before, and I did the same about Janel's story in Boston and my own.

Martineau shared with me for the first time that night how he had grown up in poverty, how he had taught his own mom how to read, and the story of how he had nearly died because of his untreated hernia when he was a child. And here he was about to start a neurology residency in the US. I had always admired Martineau greatly as a doctor, as a colleague, and as a friend. But that night at our kitchen table, I was in awe of how much he had overcome to achieve what I had taken for granted. When it was my turn to talk about my path to medicine, it seemed embarrassing to recount what I often referred to as the "struggle" in my story—deciding if I should stay in medicine or become a musician.

But we had medicine in common and now we had Janel's story in common too. It was on that night that I learned how Martineau had seen himself in Janel, how he felt called to give, in his words, "a voice to the voiceless" when he tirelessly pursued Janel's passport.

"Did I ever show you this video I have of Janel singing?" I asked Martineau.

"I don't think so," he said.

"When I think of all he went through—and all we went through with his case—seeing this video . . . It really puts it all in perspective," I said, shaking my head, choking up a bit.

"Can we watch it?" Martineau asked.

I searched through the photos on my phone and found the video. "I could never quite make out the words he's singing. Maybe you can translate for me?"

"Let's see," Martineau said.

In the video, Janel is sitting in one of his mom's white plastic lawn chairs in their house. He's wearing gray shorts and no shirt, a white towel thrown over one shoulder. His mom is sitting behind him on a bedside commode converted into a chair. She's wearing her blue, black, and yellow striped polo shirt, a black skirt, and a wide-brimmed white church hat adorned with crisscrossing strips of lace like the top of an apple pie.

As Janel puts on his Ray-Ban sunglasses from Paul Farmer, one of the neighbor's young children crawls into the open doorway behind him, which in the cell phone video appears as a luminous rectangle of midday sunlight surrounded by the lime-green walls of the one-room house. As Janel finishes adjusting his glasses, the little boy lies down on the floor in the doorway.

"Dis sou dis," I hear my voice call to Janel, complimenting him on his sunglasses. ("Ten out of ten.") It's a phrase I'd heard him say when I showed him pictures of me and my wife together.

Janel smiles widely, nodding slowly, contentedly. *"Respè, Dok,"* he says. ("Respect, Doc.")

After a pause, he begins clapping a slow, regular beat, and his mom joins his clapping. Over this beat Janel sings a spritely, syncopated tune:

Lage pwoblem yo
Nan men le Seigneur
Kit li fè
Sa li vle avek yo

After singing the verse three times through, he adds:

Pouki ou pa . . .

And then he starts again from the top.

On the second time through the song, he raises his hands with elbows bent and pumps them up and down gently as he sings, nodding his head back and forth in time with the song. At the end of this verse, he breaks from the singing to call out, *"Lage pwoblem yo!!"* as if he's announcing the next line to a group he's leading. Then he goes back to singing.

Martineau watched the video with a broad smile and laughed when Janel shouted to his invisible audience.

The video finished, and I played it again.

"So what do the words mean?" I asked Martineau. "I hear something *'pwoblem'*—is it *'pa gen pwoblem'* ('no problem')?"

"Close," Martineau said. "It's *'lage pwoblem'*—'let go of your problems.'"

"And what about the rest?" I asked.

"Can you play it one more time?" he asked.

We watched it again.

Martineau laughed again when Janel shouted out the opening line before singing it. Then he nodded slowly, his smile fading, his eyes glistening. "Wow," he said solemnly, moved. "So the words are:

"Let go of your problems
Into the hands of the Almighty

Let him do
As he wishes with them . . .

"He keeps on repeating that," Martineau said. "And then every few verses, he adds at the end 'Why don't you . . .' so it becomes:

"Why don't you
Let go of your problems
Into the hands of the Almighty
Let him do
As he wishes with them."

I remembered asking Janel and his mom if I could make a video of him singing to send to his medical team in Boston so everyone could see how well he was doing. I had imagined our colleagues at Brigham would hardly be able to believe it. This young man who had barely been able to stay awake, let alone speak. This young man who had been too weak to eat, let alone clap. This young man who nobody had thought would ever improve after his second and then third and then fourth and then fifth brain surgery. This young man who some had thought was too expensive to treat, too high-risk to treat, too unsustainable to treat.

But here he was. This young man.

He wasn't just awake and walking, eating and talking.

He was singing.

To learn more about Partners In Health and support their work to bring healthcare to the world's poorest and most in need, please visit www.pih.org.

Acknowledgments

I want to extend my gratitude first and foremost to Janel and his mother; Davidson and his father, Enel; and Pasteur Jean-Rémy and his wife, Dorotie. Their extraordinary courage and faith inspired me to write this book, and they enthusiastically encouraged me to write it so others could learn from and be inspired by them. I hope I have done justice to their stories, their journeys, and my admiration for them.

Michelle Morse and Anne Beckett are forces of nature who will not rest until every patient on this earth gets the healthcare that every human being deserves. They have taught me so much about how to do this work, about Haiti, about doing what is right—and how to do whatever it takes to make things happen.

Hermide Mercier and Joseph Lander opened their homes and their hearts to our patients, caring for them like members of their own families as they went through surgery and recovery far from home.

Ian Dunn said yes without batting an eye to what would turn out to be some of his most challenging neurosurgical cases—medically, technically, and logistically. He is a neurosurgical wizard and miracle worker who generously pushed the care of our patients in Haiti to new levels thanks to his work both inside and outside the operating room.

Mark Proctor provided wise and patient counsel as we navigated the surprising twists and turns of Davidson's case over email between Boston and Haiti. He not only provided extraordinary expert and compassionate neurosurgical care but also advocated for this care to be completely free.

Kalem Lee, Ayal Aizer, and their dedicated staff at Brigham and Women's Hospital and Dana Farber Cancer Institute provided thoughtful and compassionate care to Janel, navigating the many challenges with skill and grace despite him being one of countless patients they care for in their most challenging field of neuro-oncology.

Terri Carlson and Eileen Tye at the Ray Tye Medical Aid Foundation ensured that the foundation's mission was fulfilled with incredible generosity to help us care for our patients from Haiti.

Simona Shuster and Kerin Howard in the Brigham and Women's international office went to amazing lengths to facilitate the care of Janel and Pasteur at Brigham.

Marty Samuels trained me, hired me, and supported me to work in Haiti. His shining example of what a physician can and should be, his encouragement, and his mentorship have been a guiding light along my path to becoming a neurologist.

Marshall Wolf has generously provided the funding that has allowed us to run our neurology training program at HUM. With his support, Haiti now has three neurologists and one more in the pipeline.

One of those recently trained neurologists, François Roosevelt, has taken the lead in continuing to advance the specialty of neurology in Haiti. In his hands, the future of neurology in Haiti is bright.

Paul Farmer and Ophelia Dahl are living legends who have pioneered healthcare delivery to the world's poorest and marginalized, achieving impossible feats and avoiding failures of imagination. It has been an honor and privilege to work for and with them, and I am so grateful for their support as I stand on their giants' shoulders in this work. Ophelia has so generously and creatively helped us find solutions for some of our most challenging problems, and also somehow found time to read a draft of this book and provide incredibly helpful and perceptive insights on how to improve it. She also kindly introduced me to my wonderful agent, Jill Kneerim.

In my much-anticipated first meeting with Jill, she generously treated me to a four-hour breakfast in which she posed the perfect questions that helped me find solutions to some of the issues I had been wrestling with in my writing. She has been an inspiring mentor, incredible editor, and wonderful guide through this entire process.

Mickey Maudlin and Anna Paustenbach at HarperOne have been truly wonderful editors. They understood what I was trying to say (sometimes even better than I did), and provided thoughtful advice and inspiring encouragement to help me to say it better and more beautifully. It has been a joy and great learning experience to work with them and their team at HarperOne.

Sumita Strander, my incredibly talented research assistant, read multiple drafts of this book and gave brilliant and nuanced feedback. She is destined for an amazing career as a physician and anthropologist, and I look forward to celebrating her future contributions.

In the summer of 2017, I had lunch with a dear friend who has known me since before I was born, Rozanne Gold. Sitting under a tree in New Haven, I mentioned casually to her that I had been thinking about writing a book about some patients we had brought from Haiti to Boston for neurosurgery. She insisted I had to do it, and gently but strongly guided me to and through the process, providing inspiration, thoughtful advice, and deeply resonant reminders to remain mindful and patient at each and every step along the way.

My parents gave me a compass when I set off for college, explaining that it symbolized finding my way. I was seventeen and eager to be an adult out on my own, and the message was lost on me in the moment. Years later I would realize that they had provided me with a strong internal compass—to try to do what is right, to help others, to seek out true north. They have been extraordinarily supportive, whether I was leaving medicine for music or flying to Haiti in spite of a travel warning. I am grateful to them for the roots and wings they have selflessly provided. The compass sits on the desk at which I write these words.

My wife, Nina, has been an amazing source of encouragement, support, nourishment, and love as I worked on this book (and did the work described in this book), as she has in all aspects of our life together. She generously helped me make time and space to write, and provided thoughtful feedback on countless sentences, paragraphs, and ideas as I wrote.

Notes

Epigraph

vii   *"Hallie had been working . . ."*: Paul Auster, *4321* (New York: Henry Holt, 2017), 804.

vii   *"Our mission is . . ."*: "Our Mission at PIH," Partners In Health website, https://www.pih.org/pages/our-mission.

Chapter 1

4   *32 CT scanners per 100 million population:* World Health Organization (WHO), *Global Atlas of Medical Devices* (Geneva: World Health Organization, 2017), http://www.who.int/medical_devices/publications/global_atlas_meddev2017/en/.

4   *The earthquake devastated Haiti's overpopulated capital:* Estimates vary. See Paul Farmer, *Haiti After the Earthquake* (New York: PublicAffairs, 2011), 86; Jonathan M. Katz, *The Big Truck That Went By* (New York: Palgrave Macmillan, 2013), 70; and Amy Wilentz, *Farewell Fred Voodoo* (New York: Simon and Schuster, 2013), 181.

4   *Haiti's largest public hospital:* Farmer, *Haiti After the Earthquake*, 86, 308; and Wilentz, *Farewell Fred Voodoo*, 218.

4   *over half of US families donated:* Katz, *The Big Truck That Went By*, 69.

4   *PIH built Hôpital Universitaire de Mirebalais:* For a discussion of the development of HUM, see Paul Farmer, *To Repair the World*, ed. Jonathan Weigel (Berkeley: Univ. of California Press, 2013), 61–64; and Farmer, *Haiti After the Earthquake*, 184–86, 245.

11   *Paul Farmer—one of PIH's founders:* Farmer, *Haiti After the Earthquake*, 11, 22.

11   *About 4 billion people:* WHO/World Bank Group, *Tracking Universal Health Coverage: 2017 Global Monitoring Report* (Geneva: WHO Document Production Services, 2017), https://www.who.int /healthinfo/universal_health_coverage/report/2017/en/.

11   *PIH's mission statement:* "Our Mission at PIH," Partners In Health website, https://www.pih.org/pages/our-mission.

Chapter 2

28   *"My philosophy is what you take":* Mark Goulston, "Just Listen— Ray Tye, Boston Philanthropist, Dies at 87," *Life* (blog), *Huffington Post*, May 11, 2010, https://www.huffpost.com/entry/just-listen -ray-tye-bo_b_494116.

29   *"This is not philanthropy":* "Raymond Tye," obituary, *Lowell Sun*, March 12, 2010, http://www.legacy.com/obituaries/lowellsun/obituary .aspx?pid=140639040.

29   *the complicated story of a patient:* David Abel and Akilah Johnson, "Haiti Earthquake Survivor Dreads Departure," *Boston Globe*, February 5, 2014, https://www.bostonglobe.com/metro/2014/02/05 /four-years-after-earth-shook-haiti-survivor-remains-cambridge -hospital-and-limbo/4ZXvhm6AbRmtNtBFNbotCI/story.html #comments.

31   *Hermide grew up:* Partners In Health, "PIH Right to HealthCare Program: Whatever It Takes," *PIH Bulletin*, Summer 2007, 4–5, http://parthealth.3cdn.net/52a71b7953eecd11ec_13m6baycr.pdf.

Chapter 3

34   *The adult literacy rate:* Central Intelligence Agency Library, "The World Factbook, Central America: Haiti," last modified July 30, 2019, https://www.cia.gov/library/publications/the-world-factbook/geos /ha.html.

34   *less than a third of the population:* UNICEF, "At a Glance: Haiti: Statistics," last modified December 27, 2013, https://www.unicef.org /infobycountry/haiti_statistics.html#117.

34   *most schoolteachers are unqualified:* USAID, *Haiti: Education Fact Sheet,* January 2016, https://www.usaid.gov/sites/default/files /documents/1862/Education%20Fact%20Sheet%20FINAL%20%20 January%202016%20-2%20page.pdf.

35   *Less than a third of Haitians:* Central Intelligence Agency Library, "The World Factbook," https://www.cia.gov/library/publications/the -world-factbook/geos/ha.html.

35   *"savages and cannibals" in 1884:* Paul Farmer, *The Uses of Haiti* (Monroe, ME: Common Courage Press, 1994), 71.

35   *"unthinking black animals" in 1920:* "Haiti and Its Regeneration by the United States," *National Geographic,* December 1920, 497.

35   *"illiterate, superstitious, disease-ridden and backward":* Nina Glick-Schiller and Georges Fouron, "'Everywhere We Go, We Are in Danger': Ti Manno and the Emergence of Haitian Transnational Identity," *American Ethnologist* 17, no. 2 (1990): 329–47.

35   *"hungry, Satan-worshipping drug addicts":* Philippe Girard, *Haiti: The Tumultuous History* (New York: Palgrave Macmillan, 2010), 108, 140, 141.

35   *referred to as a "black hole":* T. D. Allman, "After Baby Doc," *Vanity Fair,* January 1989, 74–116.

36   *a "shithole" by Donald Trump:* Julie Hirschfeld Davis, Sheryl Gay Stolberg, and Thomas Kaplan, "Trump Alarms Lawmakers with Disparaging Words for Haiti and Africa," *New York Times,* January 11, 2018, https://www.nytimes.com/2018/01/11/us/politics/trump-shithole -countries.html.

37   *more than one million people injured:* Paul Farmer, *Haiti After the Earthquake,* 328.

40   *When Columbus landed:* Direct quotations of Columbus in this section come from "Letter from Columbus to Louis de Santangel," document AJ-063, American Journeys, Wisconsin Historical Society, http://www.americanjourneys.org/aj-063/index.asp; and "Journal of the First Voyage of Columbus," document AJ-062, American Journeys, Wisconsin Historical Society, http://www.americanjourneys.org /aj 062/.

40   *extinction of the Taíno:* Robert M. Poole, "What Became of the Taíno?" *Smithsonian Magazine*, October 2011, https://www.smithsonianmag .com/travel/what-became-of-the-taino-73824867/.

40   *France subsequently took control:* Discussion of Haiti's history based on Farmer, *Uses of Haiti*; Farmer, *Haiti After the Earthquake*; Girard, *Haiti: The Tumultuous History*; Jared Diamond, *Collapse* (New York: Penguin, 2006), chap. 11; Jonathan M. Katz, *The Big Truck That Went By*; and Laurent Dubois, *Haiti: The Aftershocks of History* (New York: Picador, 2012).

40   *sent the emptied slave ships:* Diamond, *Collapse*, 340.

40   *generated more revenue:* Farmer, *Uses of Haiti*, 56.

41   *estimated at three billion dollars:* Girard, *Haiti: The Tumultuous History*, 7.

41   *a population seven times higher:* Diamond, *Collapse*, 340.

41   *leading to further deforestation:* Girard, *Haiti: The Tumultuous History*, 109–10; Farmer, *Haiti After the Earthquake*, 35, 226; Farmer, *Uses of Haiti*, 109; and Katz, *The Big Truck That Went By*, 42.

41   *rural peasants migrated:* Girard, *Haiti: The Tumultuous History*, 107; and Katz, *The Big Truck That Went By*, 40.

42   *Travel Advisory for Haiti:* US Department of State, "Haiti Travel Advisory," June 11, 2019, https://travel.state.gov/content/travel/en /traveladvisories/traveladvisories/haiti-travel-advisory.html.

43   *"thumping love child of merengue, funk, and R&B":* Katz, *The Big Truck That Went By*, 197.

46   *failures of imagination:* Paul Farmer, "Countering Failures of Imagination," in *To Repair the World*.

Chapter 4

64   *truly helping Haitians or Haiti?:* Jonathan M. Katz, *The Big Truck That Went By*, 135–36. Katz writes: "By the dawn of the nation's third century, the mission trip became the template for how many Americans experienced Haiti firsthand, lending a familiar arc to their

reports: first, shock at the deprivation; then uplift by the spirit of the people; finally after the construction of a breeze-block school or a delivery of Bibles, exultation in a new closeness and humanity through faith. In remote areas, missions operated hospitals, orphanages, and schools. Thousands of missionaries went into the countryside as self-led volunteers. Many emphasized that one of their primary goals was to teach Haitians self-reliance.

"Ironically, the Haitians not only tended to harbor a faith more fervent and deeply tested than that of the missionaries, but also self-reliance beyond anything the visitors were likely to imagine. They were, after all, still alive in a country that spent 180 times less on healthcare per person than the United States, offered 83 percent fewer people adequate sanitation, and offered almost none of the basic highway, plumbing, or building infrastructure of the United States. They didn't need survival techniques, introduction to the New Testament, or even a new breeze-block school. But as in many interactions involving the wealthy North and the struggling island, community leaders didn't object, taking what they could get in the hope that the relationships would eventually yield more."

64 *10,000 non-governmental organizations:* Katz, *The Big Truck That Went By*, 50; and Amy Wilentz, *Farewell Fred Voodoo*, 176.

64 *aid groups even do harm:* Timothy T. Schwartz, *Travesty in Haiti* (Charleston, SC: BookSurge, 2008); and Laura Sullivan and Justin Elliott, "Report: Red Cross Spent 25 Percent of Haiti Donations on Internal Expenses," *Morning Edition*, NPR, June 16, 2016, https://www.npr.org/2016/06/16/482020436/senators-report-finds -fundamental-concerns-about-red-cross-finances.

65 *a sugarcoated version: Poverty, Inc.*, produced, directed, and written by Michael Matheson Miller (2014), 91 mins.; and Schwartz, *Travesty in Haiti*.

Chapter 5

67 *has been referred to as Haiti's last name:* Jean-Claude Martineau, "The Other Occupation: The Haitian Version of Apartheid," *Covert Action*

Quarterly, Spring 2005, 10–14, https://covertactionmagazine
.com/wp-content/uploads/2018/08/CAQ78.pdf.

67   *By the numbers:* "World Bank Open Data," https://data.worldbank
.org/; and Central Intelligence Agency Library, "The World Factbook,
Central America: Haiti," last modified July 30, 2019, https://www.cia
.gov/library/publications/the-world-factbook/geos/ha.html.

71   *Sweet Micky, (in)famous for:* Pras Michel, interview by Michael Martin
(host), "That Time Wyclef Jean Ran for President of Haiti," *All Things
Considered, NPR*, November 21, 2015, https://www.npr.org/2015/11/21
/456942210/that-time-wyclef-jean-ran-for-president-of-haiti; Pooja
Bhatia, "Haiti: Dancing in the Dark," *The Caravan*, June 30, 2011,
http://www.caravanmagazine.in/letters/haiti-dancing-dark; Jonathan
M. Katz, "What Happens When a Celebrity Becomes President," *The
Atlantic*, February 9, 2016, https://www.theatlantic.com/international
/archive/2016/02/haiti-michel-martelly/461991/; *Sweet Micky for
President*, directed by Ben Patterson (2015), 89 mins.; and Jonathan M.
Katz, *The Big Truck That Went By*.

74   *Protesters were demanding:* "Haiti's Prime Minister Laurent Lamothe
Resigns After Protests," *BBC* News, December 14, 2014, http://www
.bbc.com/news/world-latin-america-30468424.

Chapter 6

80   *World Health Organization website listed:* World Health Organization,
"International Travel and Health: Contraindications to Air Travel,"
https://www.who.int/ith/mode_of_travel/contraindications/en/.

88   *"The two most important days":* Quote attributed to Mark Twain,
but on the Center for Mark Twain Studies website, author Matt
Seybold writes, "If the aphorism in question indicates a sentimental,
nostalgic, or otherwise optimistic attitude towards humanity, it
probably didn't come from Twain." The original source is unknown.
Matt Seybold, "The Apocryphal Twain: 'The Two Most Important
Days of Your Life . . .'" Center for Mark Twain Studies website,
December 6, 2016, http://marktwainstudies.com/the-apocryphal
-twain-the-two-most-important-days-of-your-life/.

Chapter 8

117 *philosopher René Descartes:* Gert-Jan Lokhorst, "Descartes and the Pineal Gland," *Stanford Encyclopedia of Philosophy Archive* (Winter 2018 Edition), ed. Edward N. Zalta, last modified September 18, 2013, https://plato.stanford.edu/archives/win2018 /entries/pineal-gland/.

117 *Pineal tumors are rare:* American Brain Tumor Association, "Pineal Tumors," https://www.abta.org/tumor_types/pineal-tumors/.

120 *Haitian patient who had come to Boston:* David Abel and Akilah Johnson, "Haiti Earthquake Survivor Dreads Departure," *Boston Globe,* February 5, 2014, https://www.bostonglobe.com /metro/2014/02/05/four-years-after-earth-shook-haiti-survivor -remains-cambridge-hospital-and-limbo/4ZXvhm6AbRmt NtBFNbotCI/story.html#comments.

Chapter 10

157 *Infants born in Haiti:* All from Central Intelligence Agency Library, "The World Factbook, Central America: Haiti," last modified July 30, 2019, https://www.cia.gov/library/publications/the-world-factbook /geos/ha.html.

157 *"Sometimes compassion can be a form of contempt":* Amy Wilentz, *Farewell Fred Voodoo* (New York: Simon and Schuster, 2013), 22.

157 *"You are struck by the 'resilience'":* Ansel Herz, "How to Write About Haiti," *Crossover Dreams* (blog), *Huffington Post,* July 23, 2010, https://www.huffingtonpost.com/crossover-dreams/a-guide-for -american-jour_b_656689.html.

160 *calls a "stupid death":* Paul Farmer, "'Landmine Boy' and Stupid Deaths" (chap. 20), in *Partner to the Poor: A Paul Farmer Reader,* ed. Haun Saussy (Berkeley: Univ. of California Press, 2010), 421.

Chapter 11

170 *"the root of all that's wrong":* Tracey Kidder, *Mountains Beyond Mountains* (New York: Random House, 2003), 294.

170 *PIH defines its mission:* Paul Farmer and Gustavo Gutiérrez, *In the Company of the Poor*, eds. Michael Griffin and Jennie Weiss Block (Maryknoll, NY: Orbis Books, 2013); and Partners In Health website, "Our Mission at PIH," https://www.pih.org/pages/our-mission.

Chapter 12

189 *article I'd written about Janel:* Aaron L. Berkowitz, "All for One," *Journal of the American Medical Association* 314, no. 13 (2015): 1341–42.

Chapter 13

198 *average number of neurologists:* World Health Organization and World Federation of Neurology, *Atlas: Country Resources for Neurological Disorders* (Neurology Atlas), 2nd ed. (Geneva: World Health Organization, 2017), http://www.who.int/mental_health/neurology /atlas_second_edition/en/.

205 *TB isn't a disease of the past:* World Health Organization, *Global Tuberculosis Report 2018*, https://www.who.int/tb/publications /global_report/en/; and Paul Farmer, "The Consumption of the Poor: Tuberculosis in the Twenty-First Century" (chap. 10), in *Partner to the Poor: A Paul Farmer Reader*, ed. Haun Saussy (Berkeley: Univ. of California Press, 2010).

205 *Haiti has the highest yearly rate:* World Bank, "Incidence of Tuberculosis (per 100,000 People)," *Global Tuberculosis Report*, 2000–2017, https://data.worldbank.org/indicator/SH.TBS.INCD ?year_high_desc=false; and World Health Organization, "Haiti: Tuberculosis Profile," 2017, https://extranet.who.int/sree/Reports ?op=Replet&name=%2FWHO_HQ_Reports%2FG2%2FPROD %2FEXT%2FTBCountryProfile&ISO2=HT&LAN=EN&outtype =html.

Chapter 15

235 *In PIH's description of POSER:* Partners In Health, Unit 11, *Addressing the Social Determinants of Health Through a Program on Social and*

Economic Rights (POSER), p. 12, https://www.pih.org/sites/default/files/2017-07/PMG_U11_090811.pdf.

236   *Farmer is known to counter:* Paul Farmer refers to the "perversion of the notion of 'sustainability'—anything can be sustained for us, but almost nothing can be sustained for them" in *To Repair the World*, ed. Jonathan Weigel (Berkeley: Univ. of California Press, 2013), 42.

236   *Paul Farmer's message:* Two quotations from Paul Farmer, *Haiti After the Earthquake:* "This had been our modus operandi at Partners In Health and Zanmi Lasante for decades: to struggle to serve those right in front of us even as we struggled to think about the big picture" (p. 11); and "In many ways, however, this tension—between serving those right in front of you and seeking to reduce the longer-term risk of others ending up in front of you—has been the chief tension of my work for years. This tension has animated the work of my students, trainees, and coworkers, too, because poverty and inequality are the drivers of most of the diseases and misfortunes we see." (p. 22).

242   *a 680-page anthology:* Paul Farmer, "Human Rights and a Critique of Medical Ethics" (pt. 4), in *Partner to the Poor: A Paul Farmer Reader*, ed. Haun Saussy (Berkeley: Univ. of California Press, 2010).

245   *"They didn't get Ebola":* Office of the Secretary-General's Special Adviser on Community-Based Medicine & Lessons From Haiti, "Transcripts: Paul Farmer Commencement Address: The Keck School of Medicine of the University of Southern California," May 14, 2016, https://www.lessonsfromhaiti.org/press-and-media/transcripts/paul-farmer-commencement-address/.

Chapter 16

255   *one of Paul Farmer's medical anthropology articles:* Paul Farmer, "Bad Blood, Spoiled Milk: Bodily Fluids as Moral Barometers in Rural Haiti," *American Ethnologist* 15, no. 1 (1988): 62–83.

Chapter 18

294 *Iceland has more sheep than people*: Paul Fontaine, "Sheep Population of Iceland More Than Double Human Population," *Reykjavík Grapevine*, September 5, 2015, https://grapevine.is/news/2015/09/05 /sheep-population-of-iceland-more-than-double-human-population/.

Chapter 19

306 *Clinton described how*: "Former President Bill Clinton Class Day Speech, Harvard Commencement 2007," YouTube video, 31:47, posted by Harvard University, January 30, 2015, https://www.youtube.com /watch?v=IY4rz_ga5nM; transcript found at "Class Day Address," *Harvard Magazine*, June 6, 2007, https://harvardmagazine.com /commencement/class-day-address.

306 *Gates said he believed*: "Remarks of Bill Gates, Harvard Commencement 2007," Campus & Community, *Harvard Gazette*, June 7, 2007, https://news.harvard.edu/gazette/story/2007/06/remarks -of-bill-gates-harvard-commencement-2007/.

Chapter 20

310 *Or rather an* un*natural disaster*: Paul Farmer, "Haiti's Unnatural Disaster," *The Nation*, September 18, 2008, https://www.thenation.com /article/haitis-unnatural-disaster/; Paul Farmer, *To Repair the World*, 123; and Paul Farmer, *Haiti After the Earthquake*, 117.

Chapter 22

318 *it's not about being unlucky*: Paul Farmer, *To Repair the World*, 123.

319 *"The idea that some lives"*: Tracy Kidder, *Mountains Beyond Mountains* (New York: Random House, 2003), 294.